The Rhetoric of the Opioid Crisis

The Rhetoric of the Opioid Crisis

Rachel Sussman Kaplan

LEXINGTON BOOKS
Lanham • Boulder • New York • London

Published by Lexington Books
An imprint of The Rowman & Littlefield Publishing Group, Inc.
4501 Forbes Boulevard, Suite 200, Lanham, Maryland 20706
www.rowman.com

86-90 Paul Street, London EC2A 4NE

British Library Cataloguing in Publication Information Available

Library of Congress Cataloging-in-Publication Data Available

ISBN: 978-1-7936-4054-3 (cloth)
ISBN: 978-1-7936-4055-0 (electronic)

I am dedicating this book to my family. My children are my entire life, and I love them with my entire heart. My husband is my rock and constant source of unconditional love. My parents, who have supported me and encouraged me every step of the way, including being excellent grandparents. And to my dear friends who have been by my side for 30 years—I couldn't do life without your love and laughter. Lastly, to my mentor Dr. Fritz, who taught me so much and was a much-needed source of encouragement and kindness.

Contents

Chapter One

The Rhetoric of the Opioid Crisis and Addiction to Prescription Pain Medicine

1.1 INTRODUCTION

America has entered into uncharted territory in terms of risk parameters and challenges, unfortunately claiming more lives today than ever in recorded history. The dimensions of the opioid epidemic are immense: "An estimated 25 million adult Americans, according to the most recent data, suffer daily from pain, and 23 million others suffer from severe recurrent pain, resulting in disability, loss of work productivity, loss of quality of life, and reduced overall health status" (Meldrum, 2016, p. 1365). More than 2 million people in the United States are suffering from a substance-abuse addiction related to opioids (Center for Behavioral Health Statistics and Quality, 2016). In 2016, opioid medications in America claimed at least seventy-eight lives every day (Enomoto in U.S. Department of Health and Human Services & Centers for Disease Control and Prevention, 2016). An article entitled "Two Innovative Approaches for Treating Opioid Addiction" released in 2018 by Blue Cross and Blue Shield points out, "Each day more than 115 people die from opioid overdoses" (para 1). Opioid overdoses are fueled by the availability and usage of synthetic opioids like fentanyl and carfentanil, which are more potent than heroin (Volkow and Collins, 2017).

Modernity is the driving theoretical lens for this entire book. As Giddens reminds us, modernity is a "risk culture" where risk "becomes fundamental to the way both lay actors and technical specialists organize the social world" (2013, p. 3). The modern world is organized around managing *risk*—technical specialists like lawyers advise corporations to warn consumers when a cup of coffee is hot, and if a floor may be slick; therefore, corporations post multiple signs indicating the risk (Giddens, 2013, p. 3; Neef, 2012, p. 70). Scientists and doctors advise the Federal Drug Administration on what are safe risks for patients in terms of medical treatments and health regimens. The idea that risk is intrinsic to everyday life in modernity has implications for managing a crisis, and these implications will be further explored in future chapters of this project. This book argues through case studies of Appalachia, the smoking crisis, case studies of unethical professionals, and widespread use of pain as the fifth vital that modernity's push for fast cures and reliance on mass distribution of scientific information may have contributed to loss of human life caused by the opioid crisis. The mass-produced and disseminated information was erroneous in regard to both the smoking crisis and the opioid crisis; for instance, there was a time the doctor may have told you to smoke to cure morning sickness or sore throat or to take daily opioids for chronic pain. Ultimately, modernity seeks fast fixes and instant cures and this too contributed to people seeking a cure in the form of a pill (Harvey, 1999).

Additionally, this book explores the different agendas and rhetorical biases associated with groups involved in the crisis. In exploring rhetorical bias, ideas associated with the philosophy of communication become relevant. The philosophy of communication seeks to understand and reveal bias, and the health communication literature is written from several vantage points (Arnett and Holba, 2012, p. 6–9). There are some who view addiction as a moral failing and others who view addicts as having a neurological illness. An understanding of the rhetorical nature of science is important when reading the literature. Chapter 2 examines what constitutes a crisis and explores the rhetoric of the smoking crisis and draws connections to the opioid crisis. Chapter 3 examines the rhetorical positions of the surgeon general and high-ranking officials in the Obama administration and the Trump administration, both offering different positions of addiction as a disease versus addiction as a crime. Chapter 4 explores the role of the professional and how professionals contributed to worsening the crisis. Chapter 5 explores the role of the patient and how the patient could be misled to take opioids or empowered to say no to a doctor offering a prescription. Chapter 6 explores the family unit and the effects the opioid crisis had on children and family. Lastly, chapter 7 explores the rhetorical bias created by the pharmaceutical companies and the Sackler family.

The book argues there are several stakeholders in this crisis: doctors, hospitals, the American Pain Society, the Veterans Administration, the Sackler family, patients, and other pharmaceutical companies. This work argues each one of these groups have a different rhetorical bias and each group has contributed, some willingly, in the name of corporate profit and others inadvertently while trying to help patients.

1.2 MODERNITY AS THE THEORETICAL LENS

Modernity is the lens through which this book explores many facets of the opioid crisis. Modernity promised a commitment to progress; however, some view modernity as "a path paved by fool's gold" (Arnett, 2012, p. 1). Modernity turns away from tradition. If described as a secular religion, the "holy trinity" of modernity would be progress, efficiency, and individual autonomy (Arnett, 2012, p. 4). In modernity, "the future is constantly drawn into the present by means of the reflexive organization"; reflecting on the past and guiding practices based upon tradition is viewed as unfavorable (Giddens, 2013, p. 3). Therefore, it should come as no surprise that in modernity consumerism pervades culture, with the marketplace at the center. There is an emphasis on technology, and ever-noticeable is the shrinking gap between time and space. Giddens assigns three main characteristics to modernity: "(1) a certain set of attitudes towards the world, the idea of the world as open to transformation, by human intervention; (2) a complex of economic institutions, especially industrial production, and a market economy; (3) a certain range of political institutions, including the nation-state and mass democracy" (Giddens and Pierson, 1998, p. 94). Giddens and Pierson (1998), Giddens (2013), and Arnett (2012) indicate modernity is about progress, transformation of information, growth of the marketplace, and managing risk.

When considering the transformation of information seen in modernity, the power and influence of major institutions in modernity is notable. The works of Michel Foucault ("The Subject and Power," *Power/Knowledge*, and *The Archaeology of Knowledge*) seek to understand the relationships between power, discourse, and the institution. Foucault questions power and authority: "It is true that I became quite involved with the question of power. It soon appeared to me that, while a human subject is placed in relations of production and of signification, he is equally placed in power relations which are very complex" (1982, p. 778). Discourse, for Foucault, is not simply a linguistic concept; discourse is a way of representing knowledge through language (Hall, 2001, p. 72). Social practices are used to reinforce knowledge, and discourse constructs the topic (Hall, 2001, p. 72). Discourse, for Foucault, is not about one statement, one text, or one action from a single source; instead, discourse is characteristic of the way of thinking and the state of knowledge at one time.

The overarching way of thinking and the state of knowledge is known as an episteme (Hall, 2001, p. 73). Foucault (1980) writes, episteme is a *strategic apparatus,* which are not necessarily scientific theory but within a field of "*scientificity*" (1980, p. 197). The episteme is the "*apparatus*" which makes separation not true from the false, but what is and is not characterized as scientific (Focault, 1980, p. 197). Therefore, episteme becomes a powerful tool in deeming some piece of information scientific. The institutions that are the most powerful often have the influence to render something "scientific" and that may or may not be the case. Regarding the opioid crisis, it appears the institutions with the most power—the Veterans Administration, the American Pain Society, and the Joint Commission—drove "pain as the fifth vital sign." The quantification of pain and the recognition of pain as the fifth vital sign happened formally in 1999 when the Veterans Health Administration (VHA) instituted an initiative called "Pain as the Fifth Vital" and required medical nurses to ask patients to rate their pain on a numeric rating scale (NRS) from 0 (no pain) to 10 (intense pain) (Mularski et al., 2006, p. 607). Any mention of a pain score over four would trigger "a comprehensive pain evaluation," and opioids were often considered (Mularski et al., 2006, p. 607). Also, the Joint Commission on Accreditation of Healthcare Organizations, now called the Joint Commission (JCO), began to support the usage of an NRS for reporting pain (Morone and Weiner, 2013, p. 1729). In conclusion, the powerful institution deemed a NRS a scientific way to measure and treat pain.

Power dynamics between patient and doctor surface as Foucault explores the medical profession's power, writing that the medical profession is criticized "for an uncontrolled power over people's bodies, their health and their life and death" (Focault, 1982, p. 780). Doctors have an ethical responsibility to act in their patient's best interest and to respect the power that comes with the medical license (Miles, 2005, p. 2).

Immediacy is also relevant when considering characteristics of modernity and the opioid epidemic. Elements of immediacy exist in everything from communication to purchasing. There is a preoccupation and emphasis placed upon science to provide answers. In modernity, "the primary effect has been to emphasize the values and virtues of instantaneity (instant and fast food meals, and other satisfactions) and of disposability (cups, plates, cutlery, packaging, napkins, clothing)" (Harvey, 1999, p. 100). Modernity is a throwaway culture, "being able to throw away values, life-styles, stable relationships, and attachments to things, buildings, places, people and received ways of being and doing" (Harvey, 1999, p. 100). The disposable mentality has far-reaching consequences, including increased rates of depression and isolation, as well as divorce, and the fact that the average person in contemporary society works for a myriad number of companies. Wallerstein and Blakeslee (1990) explain divorce, by its mere existence, creates a crisis in people's lives and presents a major threat to overall feelings of personal safety while negatively impacting overall well-being (xiii–xx). Modernity brings about the reliance upon technology, disposability, and of instantaneity present challenges for those who live in a modern world. Largely as a result of turning away from tradition, turning to science for answers, revering the marketplace, along with several other characteristics discussed above, modernity is much more dynamic than any earlier type of social order. "It is a society—more technically, a complex of institutions—which, unlike any preceding culture, lives in the future, rather than the past" (Giddens and Pierson, 1998, p. 94). I seek to argue distinguishing characteristics of modernity contribute to prescription-painkiller addiction, where people turn to a pill for a quick fix as a cure for social frustrations and physical ailments.

Risk and Historical Time Period

The opioid crisis arguably began in the 1990s, with proprescribing rhetoric which encouraged physicians to take a liberal stance on prescribing opioids to their patients. Historically, opium has been used in societies for thousands of years, but what has changed are the risk parameters associated with the drug. The *risk parameters* of prescription opioid medications in modernity are now vastly greater than when opium was smoked in antiquity and the Middle Ages (Giddens, 2013). The technological advancements allowing for mass production and efficiency in distribution channels have expanded those risk parameters. The first opium use dates to the ancient civilizations of Mesopotamia located in Southwest Asia (3400 BCE), but the first surviving records of opium addiction date from the end of the eighteenth century (Kocherlakota, 2014, p. e547). The Sumerians referred to the opium poppy as "the joy plant," and the Sumerians passed "the joy plant" to the Assyrians who in turn passed it on to the Egyptians (Drug Enforcement Agency, n.d.). Opiates have been abused "since at least 300 b.c. [when] Nepenthe (Greek 'free from sorrow') helped the hero of the *Odyssey*, but widespread opium smoking in China and the Near East has caused harm for centuries" (Kosten and Haile, 2014, p. 468e).

Opium is the dried milky juice of the unripe seed capsule of the poppy, and the word opium is derived from "opos," the Greek word for juice (Van Ree et al., 1999, p. 341). Medicinal and recreational use of opium by the ancient Greeks and Romans is not well documented; however, it is believed that they were aware of the euphoric and narcotic (from the Greek word for stupor) properties of opium (Van Ree et al., 1999, p. 341). It is suspected that the Greeks and Romans also knew that opium could be applied for pain relief and dysentery (Van Ree et al., 1999, p. 341). Furthermore, there are suggestions that the "opium poppy was cultivated in Persia back to the end of the third millennium, and Arabic doctors prescribed opium often. Arabic traders brought opium from the eighth century AD on, first to the East, to India and China, and later to Europe" (Van Ree et al., 1999, p. 341). The Mohammedan prohibition of drinking alcohol and the banning of tobacco smoking in China may have contributed to the spread of opium (Van Ree et al., 1999, p. 341).

"The Silk Road" is a series of interconnected routes that connected Europe to China from 200 BC to 300 BC, and opium was one of the products traded along the Silk Road (Drug Enforcement Agency, n.d.). However, when Britain controlled the East India Company, the company began smuggling Indian opium to China (Drug Enforcement Agency, n.d.). Once the Indian opium entered the Chinese market, the demand soared; it was a contributing factor to the Opium Wars of the 1800s, and addiction rates among Chinese citizens were noted in medical literature (Van Ree et al., 1999, p. 341).

In China in the early twentieth century, "many Chinese regarded opium as a panacea for illnesses, ailments, and other maladies. Although it was merely an analgesic that blocked the neural transmission of pain from the affected area to the brain, most people associated the cessation of pain with a medicinal 'cure.' Many such people acquired the habit, and the result was widespread opium addiction" (Slack, 2001, p. 40). In the 1930s, opium smoking had become a part of the Chinese culture: "Funerals, weddings, or feasts, on any occasion when many guests are invited, a number of rooms is prepared for smoking with beds, pipes, lamps and opium provided for all smokers. This is done openly. Opium is provided as a matter of course, just as is wine" (Slack, 2001, p. 41). Opium smoking in China was a sign of refinement and class in the 1900s. Chinese homes displayed ornate pipes for smoking and having more than one pipe was a symbol of family wealth (Slack, 2001, p. 41). Quickly, people became addicted to the opium and social problems followed including theft, robbery, prostitution, and parents were not adequately caring for children (Slack, 2001). Memoirs and interviews of people who lived during the Republic era reported lower-class men often sold their wives and children to satisfy their cravings for opium (Slack, 2001, p. 48).

The Chinese government, the Anti-Opioid Association, the National Christian Council of China, and the Anti-Narcotics Commission all worked together to lessen the effects of the Chinese opium crisis by educating the Chinese people about opium dangers, teaching Chinese farmers alternative farming practices to grow other crops instead of opium poppies, and outlawing opium in certain forms from society (Slack, 2001).

In the United States in the mid-1800s, many Chinese people began to work for railroads and in the Gold Rush and brought the habit of opium smoking with them. Opium dens sprang up in San Francisco's Chinatown and spread eastward to New York around 1850 (Martin, 2012). Americans seeking to smoke opium hired Chinese attendants to prepare pipes for them, and Chinese people usually ran American opium dens (Martin, 2012). According to Martin (2012), China was the primary source of the chandu (potent opium for smoking) and its unusual paraphernalia. For numerous reasons, opium's association with Chinese people remained after opium became widely smoked among non-Chinese. By 1905, the U.S. Congress banned opium, and the United States relied upon police raids to shut down opium dens (Martin, 2012). By 1958, the last opium den in the United States was closed (Tosches, 2002). The last opium den was located in Chinatown in New York, and Lau, a Chinese immigrant ran the den (Tosches, 2002). Lau was arrested and prosecuted, and that was the last known opium den in America (Tosches, 2002).

In this historical moment, the United States is amid an opioid crisis killing the young and the old. Opium dens are no longer the problem; in this historical moment, prescription opioids from doctors are the primary source of the issue because of overprescribing behaviors that are not in accordance with "appropriate medical use of opiates" (Ballantyne, 2007, p. 811). Federal and state governments are spending unprecedented amounts of money to try to combat the problem, and workplaces and health insurers are incurring great economic costs as well. Birnbaum et al. (2011) report that "the total societal costs of prescription opioid abuse in 2007 were calculated to be $55.7 billion, of which lost workplace productivity contributed $25.6 billion, healthcare costs contributed $25.0 billion, and criminal justice costs accounted for the remaining $5.1 billion" (p. 1). The aforementioned statistics make it clear that the United States is amid a crisis. The risks associated with mass production of opioids and the idea that society can "progress" and no longer feel pain were facets of the crisis that the lens of modernity helps to illuminate.

Health communication campaigns are being constructed to educate the public and health professionals on the issue. "Health communication operates within a very complex environment in which encouraging and supporting people to adopt and sustain healthy behaviors, or policymakers and professionals to introduce new policies and practices, or healthcare professionals to provide adequate and culturally competent care are never easy tasks" (Schiavo, 2013, p. xxiii). There have been successful campaigns targeted to dentists, emergency room doctors, and all clinicians about the need to reduce opioid prescriptions. The New York City Department of Health and Mental Hygiene (DOHMH) sponsored a health campaign targeting doctors in Staten Island, New York, and as part of this two-month campaign where doctors received one-on-one training about three main points; (1) a three-day supply of opioids is usually sufficient for acute pain, (2) avoid prescribing opioids for chronic non-cancer pain, and (3) avoid high-dose opioid prescriptions, and some improvement was made (Kattan et al., 2016). The results were positive for the campaign, "Among 866 healthcare providers visited, knowledge increased for all 3 recommendations ($P<.01$). After the campaign, the overall prescribing rate decreased similarly in Staten Island and other New York City counties (boroughs), but the high-dose prescribing rate decreased more in Staten Island than in other boroughs ($P<.01$)" (Kattan et al., para 3, 2016). Ohio, which had the fifth highest overdose rate in the country, has acted to quickly improve opioid safety (Penm et al., 2017). In 2011, the Governor's

Cabinet Opiate Action Team constructed a multifaceted approach including but not limited to tracking opioid prescriptions, reducing opioid prescriptions, and educating professionals. One of the campaigns constructed was entitled "Sometimes We Just Have to Say No" and this campaign targeted pharmacists and trained them on how to have difficult conversations with the public who are seeking inappropriate opioid prescriptions (Penm et al., 2017). Also, this campaign directed pharmacists to provide information about opioid abuse treatment programs to the public. As a result of a multifaceted approach there was a substantial reduction of overdose deaths in Ohio.

Former U.S. Surgeon-General Vivek Murthy spearheaded an effort to construct a report to bring awareness of the crisis to community members and physicians. Changing mindsets of the doctors who prescribe opioids is just as important as asking the patients who are prescribed them to demand an alternative medication. The various parties involved in the crisis all have a different agenda and their rhetorical bias should be explored. Pharmaceutical companies launched aggressive marketing campaigns and encouraged physicians to prescribe. The Centers of Disease Control and Prevention (CDC) encouraged physicians to stop overprescribing opiods. Both messages were being communicated all while local police departments and hospitals were overwhelmed with overdoses. Thomas Kuhn's (1970) *The Structure of Scientific Revolutions* illustrates the rhetorical nature of science through the concept of paradigm shifts. Paradigm shifts, according to Kuhn (1970), occur when a set of facts is constructed to persuade people to abandon old models or ways of thinking for a new way of thinking. Kuhn's (1970) work encourages thought into why scientific opinions change over time, the process of abandoning old paradigms, and the persuasive nature of attracting people to adopt the new paradigm. Kuhn's (1970) work is important when examining shifts in the scientific literature. For example, in the 1990s a set of rhetorical facts were constructed to convince doctors that opioids for chronic pain were best practice, but in the early 2000s a new set of rhetorical facts were constructed that opioids were not the best treatment for chronic pain and cause opioid addictions. This book documents the shift from proprescribing literature to conservative opioid prescribing as the dominant paradigm.

In addition to paradigm shifts, this book examines the role of personal responsibility and personal flourishing (chapter 5). The role of personal flourishing is explored through the lens of Aristotle, but Schrag (1999) serves as a brief introduction to the role of the individuals' responsibility in the opioid crisis. In the introduction to *The Self after Postmodernity*, Calvin Schrag reminds readers that people are not faced with a unitary self-portrait but a "curiously diversified portrait," and it is important to understand yourself (1999, p. 1). In other words, in current society, people identify themselves through multiple roles—as, for example, mother, father, child, or teacher, or as perpetually disabled, drug abuser, or corrupt professional. Schrag elucidates this point by quoting Socrates's "know thyself" dictum and its corollary, "The unexamined life is not worth living." But self-examination may not be of the utmost priority. A recent article in the *New York Times* discusses a countrywide trend: "In Ohio, fatal overdoses more than quadrupled in the last decade, and by 2007 had surpassed car crashes as the leading cause of accidental death, according to the Department of Health" (Tavernise, 2011, p. 1). Prescription-pain-medicine addiction is a major problem across the nation. The CDC released a report with alarming statistics: "The unprecedented rise in overdose deaths in the United States parallels a 300% increase since 1999 in the sale of these strong painkillers. These drugs were involved in 14,800 overdose deaths in 2008, more than cocaine and heroin combined" (United States, Department of Health and Human Services, Centers for Disease Control and Prevention, 2011, p. 4).

Many unsuspecting people walk into doctors' offices and leave with a litany of addictive prescription medications. A report released by New York State Attorney General Eric Schneiderman finds that "the rapid spread of prescription-drug use and abuse in New York State . . . shows that prescriptions for oxycodone, a widely prescribed narcotic painkiller, rose by 82 percent from 2007 to 2010" (Kleinfield, 2012). In 2014, three Pittsburgh doctors were arrested for illegally prescribing opioid drugs to patients. Attorney General Kathleen Kane said, "The evidence in this case will show that these physicians believed they were above the law and what's worse, they allegedly preyed upon drug-addicted patients to line their own pockets" (Kane in Born, 2014, p. 1). The professional commitment to the Hippocratic Oath of *do no harm* was abandoned for personal gain. Surgeon General Murthy, in the foreword to his report, encourages readers to engage in a paradigmatic shift for societal change and understand addiction as a neurological condition and not a moral failing (U.S. Department of Health and Human Services & Centers for Disease Control and Prevention, 2016, p. v). Murthy (2016) encourages both physicians and community members to take into account that addiction is a disease.

1.3 LITERATURE

Catt (2012) examines the problems associated with the discourse surrounding medical treatment of depression with antidepressants. In examining this discourse, he focuses on the "biologism that underwrites this worldview" (2012, p. 82), referring to the often-overlooked body-mind connection. Catt (2012) asserts that while problems are often treated as either a mind issue or a body issue, usually a problem is both. Additionally, he discusses the problems with the "psychopharmacological *Weltanschauung* that grounds the antidepressant myth in egocentric culture" (p. 82)—basically, if there is a problem, there is a pharmacological solution. Catt (2012) explains, "The worldview created around depression is a paradigm exemplar of a semiotic sphere. It is a constructed reality. It consists of not one ideology but a coded system of systems of ideas built upon myths and sustained by ongoing preconscious narratives" (p. 83). There is a litany of television commercials for depression medications, all constructed of a series of coded systems.

The coded systems are the person's affect, dress, energy, and level of engagement with others. One ad, for the depression medicine Cymbalta, shows a woman solemnly sitting on a chair when her dog brings a ball to play, but the women is lacking the energy to play. The point of the commercial is that depression hurts more than just the depressed person and also deprives the person suffering from depression of the simple pleasures in life. The woman begins to take the medicine, the sun instantly shines, and she and the dog are back to playing at the park. Also pictured in that same commercial is a woman too tired and sore to get out of bed to enjoy the day, but she easily awakens to a new day after the medication. The commercial does not focus on the element of exercise that the woman is getting while playing at the park with the dog or the abundance of social interactions that she seems to have while engaged in the activity. Rather, the solution is only the pill.

Catt refers to the social tactics that construct a worldview as *Zeitgeist*. *Zeitgeist* is a term that Georg Hegel refers to in *Lectures on Philosophy of History*, when he uses the German "*der Geist seiner Zeit*." *The Hegel Dictionary* explains this as "no man can surpass his own time, for the spirit of his time is also his own spirit" (Magee, 2010, p. 262). I have interpreted this to mean that, within the aforementioned context, we are living in a time of quick fixes and drugs advertised similarly to candy, cereal, and soda. Additionally, the "spirit" of the time is plagued with addiction. Therefore, this coded system leads people to a simple problem/one-step solution ideology. The commercial serves as a form of a health narrative in that it is constructed with the mere goal of a pharmacological solution.

The health narrative serves five main functions: sense-making, asserting control, transforming identity, warranting decisions, and building community (Thompson et al., 2003, p. 10). The commercial attempts to assert control and make sense of a complex, nuanced health issue. The problem is reduced to a three-minute problem with a simple fix. I will stress that nonspecific pain is very similar to depression; as Bair et al. (2003) report, "Depression and pain share biological pathways and neurotransmitters, which has implications for the treatment of both concurrently" (p. 2433). Nonspecific pain occurs when a patient reports pain usually in the back or neck. Nonspecific pain cannot be seen on an MRI, X-ray, or blood test. "The patient filters nerve sensations from the body through cultural, emotional, and personal lenses to identify if the pain exceeds the patient's ability to tolerate the pain and the need to access treatment," and the patient reports the sensation using a scale of zero to ten to the doctor (Wacholtz et al., 2007, p. 147). This is akin to depression, which is rarely seen on a brain scan. There is often no physical proof of depression, but a recent article describes current clinical trials to pinpoint specific areas in the brain affected by depression; however, these findings are inconclusive and preliminary and have not yet been replicated (*Brain Scan May Predict Best Depression Treatment*, 2013, p. x). Ordinarily, the doctor takes the subjective symptoms the patient reports and formulates the diagnosis. "The physics of our century has taught us that there are limits to what we can measure" (Gadamer, 1996, p. vii). Gadamer reminds us that modernity has afforded many tools to doctors to get *objective* data; however, there are just some things that cannot be quantified.

There is an even more compelling reason to believe that depression and pain are bedfellows: "On average, 65% of patients with depression experience one or more pain complaints, and depression is present in 5% to 85% (depending on the study setting) of patients with pain conditions" (Bair et al., 2003, p. 2441). Medical Doctors Michael Sullivan and Joyce D'Eon (1990) researched the relationship between depression, pain, and catastrophizing: "Catastrophizing is a cognitive process characterized by a lack of confidence and control and an experience of negative outcomes" (260). Clinical and experimental pain research concludes, "that catastrophizing thoughts are related to reports of increased pain and depression" (263).

This further illustrates the body-mind connection stressed by Catt and Gadamer. *The Handbook of Health Communication* reinforces this concept by making "explicit that there are psychological and spiritual components of health integrated with physical components" (Thompson, 2003, p. 13). The body-mind connection, along with a holistic view of health, is vital in understanding pain and how pain can be intensified with feelings of depression and sadness.

1.4 LANGUAGE AND REALITY

How someone speaks about his or her health and the pain he/she experiences is relevant to understanding the Other. Discourse theory "is a theory of language and communication, a perspective on social interaction and an approach to knowledge construction across history, societies, and cultures" (Wetherell et al., 2001, p. 1). More importantly, discourse theory examines "social phenomena as structured semiotically by codes and rules" and meaning as "socially constructed by institutions" (Best and Kellner, 1997, p. 26). The institutions that are involved in the problem of addiction are hospitals, doctor's offices, clinics, families, and communities plagued by countless victims losing their lives. Discourse theory is important when studying health communication because what is said about a condition, how a patient describes his or her health, and how the doctor responds to the patient's concerns all shape the patient's construct of reality. "Studying discourse and medicine together brings us to encounter culture as discursively constituted" (Wilce, 2009, p. 199). Discourse and culture work symbiotically to understanding the Other and their point of view.

In 1966, Berger and Luckmann understood how one's reality is constructed through language. Berger and Luckmann (1966) defined social construction through the dialectal. In other words, "social constructions of reality are mediated through linguistic expression articulated among people and communities," and nowhere is that more apparent than in Appalachia, with the way prescription-drug abuse has plagued families for generations. Justin Jenkins, a resident of Ohio, is twenty years old and a second-generation OxyContin addict; he has been sentenced to a rehabilitation program in lieu of prison. The problem runs deep through his family: his mother died of an overdose when he was ten, his aunt is an addict, and his grandfather is in prison for dealing. Justin says, "It all boils down to getting high. It messed up my whole life. I'm done with it. I'm not doing it anymore" (qtd. in Tavernise, 2011). *The Handbook of Health Communication* further highlights the familial and community semiotic connection: a "socially shared health-related narrative, is among the most powerful forms of symbolic construction" (Thompson, 2003, p. 10).

1.5 WORLDVIEWS/PARADIGMS

The worldview created around nonspecific pain is similar to that of depression because "communication grounds consciousness" (Catt, 2012, p. 89). Just as Catt asserts, there is a lot to be depressed about in the modern world; high unemployment, lack of financial stability, and high rates of divorce. There is also a tremendous number of reasons to feel pain; poverty, lack of opportunity, and family instability are just a few. Giddens (2013) outlines the problems of modernity: "Science, technology, and expertise" play a prominent role in the "sequestration of experience," and the idea that science has a greater role in society than ethics and morals (9). Day-to-day social life becomes sequestered from what it meant in its natural state and is replaced with mediated technologies. "The mad, the criminal and the seriously ill are physically sequestered" and sequestration for many other "average" people is eradicating direct contact with events and situations that link life span to broad issues of morality and finitude (Giddens, 2013, p. 150). Another problem causing pain to manifest both physically and mentally is "personal meaninglessness"—the feeling that life has nothing to offer (Giddens, 2013, p. 9). Life becomes painful as one is sequestered or removed from experiences, and, as Catt (2012) puts it, "coping is the new ethos" (p. 100).

"Pain is a multidimensional construct that is influenced by biological, psychological, and social factors" (Melzack quoted in Wachholtz, 2011, p. 145). Deacon (2013) explains the biomedical model focuses on diagnosing an illness and treating it pharmacologically, and this is in contrast to the biopsychosocial model, which focuses on biological, psychological, and social factors. The biopsychosocial model focuses on a body-mind connection and considers cultural and social factors and encourages consultation with multiple health professionals, diet, exercise, cognitive behavioral therapy, family counseling, and overall holistic wellness (Deacon, 2013).

Catt (2012) reminds us "A worldview is not necessarily directly known to a person" (83); rather, it is the everyday discourse surrounding the worldview that makes it real. Appalachia, which consists of Ohio, Kentucky, and West Virginia, faces extremely high rates of overdose of prescription pain medicine in the United States. As proof of this, in 2010 in Portsmouth, Ohio, "Nearly 1 in 10 babies born last year in this Appalachian county tested positive for drugs" (Tavernise, 2011, para 3). Parts of Appalachia provide prime examples of how discourse shapes worldviews and how discourse shapes reality; this is seen as the problem plaguing families and communities. "By illness, I mean the conscious experience of sickness. Sickness refers to what is likely to be perceived as an undesirable change in a person's health condition. This may be a minor disharmony or a more serious disembodied communication with the world. It may include any number of real or imaginary things from injury, pain, emotional suffering or hallucinations" (Catt, 2012, p. 9). Portsmouth, Ohio, was once a booming industrial town, but now it is filled with vacant storefronts and low-income people. The vacant store windows have become *picture memorials* to those who have lost their lives to drug abuse, especially the young generations (Tavernise, 2011). Additionally, a common sight is mothers whose children have died from overdoses of prescription painkillers picketing clinics who give out these prescriptions.

David Morris is a writer and scholar, and an emeritus professor of literature at the University of Virginia. The focus of his work is pain and its various manifestations. He has written several books, including *The Culture of Pain* (1991) and *Illness and Culture in the Postmodern Age* (1998). Morris is well-respected by the medical community as he was asked to speak at conferences including the American Academy of Pain Management. David Morris (1998) explains that illness is "situated at the crossroads of biology and culture" (p.

71). Even more insightful may be his claim that "illness is a fluid process that changes as we change, enigmatic, insubordinate, and subjective . . . and alters under the influence of nonmedical events from divorce to climate change" (Morris, 1998, p. 5). More simply put, the medical community may offer pills before truly understanding the entire cultural-social problem, only treating symptoms and never touching the main issue. "Quite simply, treatment of the body is not a logical first choice for a cultural-social-psychological problem, which is to say communicative illness" (Catt, 2012, p. 82). Bair et al. (2003) explain that doctors may be missing that pain could stem from a communicative illness in that "physical complaints may be due to amplification of chronic physical disease and remain medically unexplained after extensive workup. As a result, providers frequently assess for physical causes of pain and treat medically instead of exploring the pain symptoms in a broader, biopsychosocial context" (p. 245). *Interrogating Gendered Pathologies* (2020) further supports exploring pain in a broader biopsychosocial context with much attention on gender. Specifically, Frost and Eble (2020) look at illness, pain, and disease through the lens of pathology. Frost and Eble (2020) define pathology as "the process by which causes and symptoms of diseases are determined—clearly has rhetorical, social, and cultural components that are just as significant" (p. 3). Frost and Eble (2020) note "Biomedicine is gendered" and mainstream medicine considers the male body the standard (p. 7). In general, a woman's pain does not receive the same attention as a man's pain, "Nationwide, men wait an average of 49 minutes before receiving an analgesic for acute abdominal pain. Women wait an average of 65 minutes for the same thing" (Fassler 2015 in Frost and Eble 2020). Hernández and Dean (2020) make the point much attention in the research has been devoted to the gender of the physician but not that of the patient. Emily Martin's research from 1987 to 1988 explores the upon ways various medical and scientific discourses converge to construct the female body as a (failed) machine (Martin in Hernández and Dean, 2020). Therefore, the treatment of pain, the cultural constructs of gender, and biopsychosocial model are pertinent considerations for this book. The idea that "time is money" is relevant; it is a timely endeavor to converse with patients regarding underlying issues which may be causing pain in one's life. The biomedical approach entails prescribing a medication to cure an ailment, it may be time efficient, but not cure the actual problem. In short, biopsychosocial considerations are often left unexamined, as these issues are not measurable in a modern biomedical model.

1.6 HEALTH AS A BUSINESS

In modernity, the prevailing view is that the marketplace can offer a solution to just about any problem. When one opens a magazine or turns on the television, there are ads for drugs to cure all types of aliments, including restless leg syndrome, acne, dry mouth, halitosis, depression, and dry eyes, as well as a litany of drugs and surgical options promising to end the battle with obesity. Yet Gadamer realizes that "Health is not something that can be simply made or produced" (p. vii). But in modernity, health is a product. "Americans in particular have a remarkable confidence in anything that is made to appear scientific and technologically advanced. It also fits the egocentric *Weltanschauung* to focus not on the social aspects of illness, and not on the communicative relationship of a self and its world, but on the individual's responsibility for action. A self who cannot seem to act is in need of a fix" (Catt, 2012, p. 97). The interesting fact remains that the drugs that are prescribed to fix the problem may not be effective in their intended use: "a recent study from Denmark where opioids are prescribed liberally for chronic pain, demonstrated worse pain, higher healthcare utilization, and lower activity levels in opioid-treated patients compared to a match cohort of chronic-pain patients not using opioids, suggesting that even if a marginal number of patients benefit, the overall population does not when opioids are prescribed liberally" (Erikson et al., 2006, p. 172–179). The psychological component of pain cannot be overlooked: "A number of psychological factors have been shown empirically to alter a patient's pain experience. Emotional status can have a significant impact on a patient's pain experience" (Wachholtz et al., 2011, p. 145). The pharmacological industry thoroughly understands the egocentric tendency of the physician too: "Opioid analgesics remain the mainstay of pharmacologic treatment for acute and chronic pain. However, the risks for misuse and development of addiction have raised concerns for clinicians, public health specialists, and the community at large" (Wachholtz et al., 2011, p. 145).

The fact remains that if patients continually visit their doctors for prescriptions, the doctor is receiving money for the visit and other "treatments" performed. Additionally, the pill may be pushed due to the vast promotions executed by the pharmacological industry: "Expansion of opioid therapy for patients who might benefit more from nondrug interventions or alternate drugs, without consideration of the accompanying risks of opioids, is based on pharmaceutical promotion" (Manchikanti, 2007, p. 417). There is a clear connection with the escalation of the prescribing of opioids and the aggressive marketing campaign of OxyContin, which encouraged doctors to be proactive with chronic-pain patients. In fact, the *New England Journal of*

Medicine reports "escalations parallel an increase by a factor of 10 in the medical use of opioids since 1990" (Okie, 2010, p. 1982). The marketing blast was first launched in the nineties, but the problem persists. In the fall of 2013, when the FDA approved the powerful prescription pain-relieving drug Zohydro, a coalition of more than forty health care, consumer, and addiction-treatment groups wrote a letter to the FDA commissioner saying, "In the midst of a severe drug epidemic fueled by overprescribing of opioids, the very last thing the country needs is a new, dangerous, high-dose opioid" (Smith, 2014, p. 1). Another side of the argument of the approval of Zohydro is brought to light: "The problem is, it costs a lot of money bringing a drug through clinical trials and then bringing it to market," says Anderson, past president of the Washington chapter of the American College of Emergency Physicians. "You have to anticipate (the drug company) being able to market and get its money back" (Smith, 2014, p. 1). Dr. Anderson ended his interview by stating, "Put more of this kind of drug out on the street and I'll see more overdoses related to this, no question" (Smith, 2014, p. 1). This reverts back to modernity. Is the profit incentive of the pharmacological industry of greater concern than human life?

Transforming medicine into a profit-generating entity can become problematic: "Healthy is used to characterize what is found in nature," yet it is marketed as if health were a candy or shampoo (Thompson, 2003, p. 13). Gadamer realizes that "the institutionalization of science into a business belongs to the larger context of economic and social life in the industrial age" (Gadamer, 1996, p. 17). This ultimately leads to a lack of patient autonomy because "virtues of accommodation and adjustment to such rational forms of organization are correspondingly cultivated, the autonomy of the formation of judgment and of action according to one's own judgment are correspondingly neglected" (1996, p. 17). The professional judgment of a doctor may be clouded by economic incentive. Some doctors have become the modern-day drug dealer for those addicted to opioids: "Street drug users can obtain prescription opioids for pain and/or withdrawal therapy from doctors or pharmacies 57.9 percent of the time, but also obtain them from dealers 41.9 percent of the time" (Davis and Johnson, 2008, p. 10). The appropriate way to prescribe opioids for pain is to conduct a functional-goal analysis. A functional-goal analysis involves a conversation between the doctor and the patient whereby they come up with a list of "three goals that the patient would be able to accomplish if they experienced less pain" (Wachholtz et al., 2011, p. 145). What makes this treatment modality different is that "the provider and patient do not wait until the patient is pain-free to begin behavioral activation, but it occurs on the first visit" (Wachholtz et al., 2011, p. 145). This approach takes a great deal of time, and time is money; additionally, this approach takes into account the psychological effects of social isolation and estrangement from daily activity. The idea behind this strategy is to return the patient back to daily activity rather than a total alleviation of the pain. The functional-goal approach is not widely used because many doctors who are prescribing the opioids are not trained.

Diversion is defined as "the transfer of a prescription drug from a lawful to an unlawful channel of distribution or use" (Inciardi et al., 2007, p. 172). Diversion occurs through multiple ways, "including: the illegal sale of prescriptions by physicians and what are referred to on the street as 'loose' pharmacists; 'doctor shopping' by individuals who visit numerous physicians to obtain multiple prescriptions; theft, forgery, or alteration of prescriptions by healthcare workers and patients" (Inciardi et al., 2007, p. 172).

An extreme example of doctors' abuse of prescription opioids is Ronald McIver, a former doctor at the Pain Therapy Center in Greenwood, South Carolina. He is now a prisoner in North Carolina "serving 30 years for drug trafficking" (Rosenberg, 2007, p. 1). He treated his patients aggressively with high doses of OxyContin. McIver's reckless prescribing led to lethal dosage amounts; an insurance agent monitoring the claims filed by McIver on a patient said, "The amounts were incredible; it jumped out in my face. He was either selling them or taking so much he couldn't live" (qtd. in Rosenberg, 2007, p. 1). Two days later, the Drug Enforcement Agency (DEA) was involved and showed up with an administrative subpoena. The information collected included messy offices filled with manila envelopes stuffed with patient records and receipts and used syringes overflowed their storage box. After a long trial, it was revealed that McIver had concerns, some patients paid cash despite having insurance, and patients went to great extremes to act as if they did not know one another. Despite his concerns, McIver continued to practice *medicine* from his clinic until the DEA's involvement.

1.7 THE ENIGMA OF HEALTH

Hans-Georg Gadamer, the author of *The Enigma of Health*, was a German philosopher born in Marburg in 1900, and he lived to the age of 102. Gadamer grew up with a father who was a pharmacist, and his mother died when he was young. His father valued strongly the natural sciences and not the humanities, but Gadamer chose to study the humanities. Gadamer was a student of the Marburg School and learned from both Husserl and Heidegger. Unlike Heidegger, Gadamer was neither a member nor supporter of the Nazi Party (Dostal, 2002). Gadamer, as a philosopher, had insight into health and the human condition.

He wrote *The Enigma of Health*, a collection of essays discussing multiple aspects of health. Gadamer makes it clear that this book is not simply for doctors; rather, it is for ordinary people who will inevitably become patients. Gadamer writes about health through the paradigm of shared responsibility; the responsibility is placed upon the individual, the science community, the patient, and society. There are limits to measurement and in Gadamer's opinion this alone "merits strong hermeneutical interest" (1996, p. vii). Later, Gadamer (1996) makes the point that modern science's goal of objectification and constant measurement is a "violent estrangement from ourselves" (70). Gadamer notes that health cannot only be treated "solely from the perspective of science" (p. viii). He says that people begin to think about health and their personal well-being in the absence of health; in other words, health escapes our attention.

Gadamer leads the reader through the history of "positive" science, which effectively left metaphysics behind and in turn brought about philosophical positivism. Positivism is based on quantification, numbers, and statistics. In 1982, Halfpenny identified three main philosophical positions in classical positivism: scientism, empiricism, and naturalism (May and Mumby, p. 18). Scientism is a theory of historical development in which improvements in knowledge are both the motor of historical progress and the source of social stability. Empiricism is a theory of knowledge available to mankind; it is that of science, grounded in observation. Naturalism is a unity-of-science thesis, according to which all sciences can be integrated into a single natural system.

In Gadamer's *Truth and Method*, he explains, "What makes coming to an understanding possible is language which provides the 'Mitte'" (the middle, the middle ground, the place where understanding, as we say, takes place) (1989, preface, p. 3). Unlike Hobbes, Gadamer does not think understanding is reached via a "social contract" that can be agreed to in advance, nor does he believe it is reached through psychological means such as empathy and sympathy. Rather, Gadamer stresses that understanding is achieved through a "common willingness of the participants in conversation to lend themselves to the emergence of something else" and the "Sache or subject matter which comes to presence and presentation in the conversation" (1989, p. xvii). Therefore, in both *Truth and Method* and *The Enigma of Health* (1996), there needs to be a willingness of both parties—in this case, doctors and patients—to lend themselves to a conversation with the emergence of the "sache" at the surface. The phrase "living body and life" presents the "inseparability of the living body and life itself"—there is an ontological component to body and soul. In this line of thinking, there is an absolute inseparability, as it would be impossible to live in a body without a soul. This view is in contrast to the external view on the world created through modern science. In an external view of the world, one is encouraged to "observe, among all its various phenomena, our own bodily experience" (Gadamer, 1996, p. 71). Gadamer questions: "Is it possible to be connected once again with our own lived experience, or must the experience of one's own individuality be lost irrevocably in the context of modern data banks and new technology?" (Gadamer, 1996, p. 72). Additionally, the idea that "the body cannot be treated without at the same time treating the soul" originally arises from Plato's *Phaedrus*. In Germany, one who is unwell literally says, "*Es fehlt mir etwas*," which translates to "I am lacking in something" (Gadamer, 1996, p. 73). Gadamer asks what we can learn from these etymological considerations. The state of being healthy or, in other words, the state of being whole "poses ontological primacy" and is the natural condition of life. When one is lacking in something it may take a significant amount of time to surface, yet the modern doctor formulates a diagnosis in a very different way. To determine a diagnosis, the doctor will question the patient directly and ask the patient to "testify to the fact that being ill involves a disturbance whose cause remains concealed" (Gadamer, 1996, p. 130). Gadamer remarks that a modern doctor may feel that a standard question inquiry would be sufficient to uncover the problem but an "experienced doctor knows that such a method can only provide guidelines and provide a preliminary overview of medical findings" (1996, p. 130). In modernity, profit and efficiency are defining characteristics. Doctors sometimes skip sufficient inquiry, and this can lead to catastrophic outcomes. Abraham, Naik, and Street (2012) discuss shared decision making in a clinical setting. Abraham, Naik, and Street (2012) provide an example that highlights shared decision-making between doctor and patient can be a matter of life and death; a 66-year-old man with a history of colon cancer and polyps who missed his appointment for a colonoscopy. When the doctor asked him why he stated that he was never asked if he was physically able to perform the preparation for the procedure on his own. The patient skipped his colonoscopy because the prescribing doctor never bothered to ask the patient if he needed any help in getting to the procedure. Abraham, Naik, and Street (2012) conclude shared decision-making is a necessity, "A shift towards a meaningful dialogue between patients and physicians requires us to acknowledge uncertainties associated with a clinical decision and ensure that patients' health beliefs are acknowledged and included in the decision-making" (p. 825). Patients feel a sense of agency and responsibility when they are involved in their health-related decisions, clinician-patient communication can improve health by empowering patients to be active, capable agents in managing their health (Street et al., 2009).

The experience of health is similar to the process of falling asleep; it is marked "by a particularly mysterious and obscure character" (Street et al., 2009, p. 131). Gadamer (1996) asserts health is a strong but concealed harmony, and as soon as a physical discomfort surfaces the harmony is disturbed.

The idea that health is something that most people only consider once it is missing contributes to the *Zeitgeist* of the modern world. Modernity brings with it a break with tradition and highlights the holy trinity of "progress, efficiency and individual autonomy," thus further disconnecting the individual with the community and the self (Arnett, 2012, p. 4). The pharmacological gestalt that Isaac Catt explains pervades all aspects of medicine form the idea of what an illness is and how it should be treated. In a world where waiting around is viewed as a person who is unwilling to engage in a fix is seen as lazy, yet modernity pushes the ideas of "fixing" the ailment even if it means creating two new problems: addiction and dependency. The meaningful nature of work and family becomes shattered when addiction is introduced, and the downward spiral so often seen in chronic-pain patients is viewed through the paradigmatic lens of a problem that science can fix.

Morris (1998) asserts the illnesses that exist in postmodernity are different from the illnesses that plagued people 50 years ago; chronic fatigue syndrome and restless leg syndrome are just a few new illnesses. Morris (1998) also points out traditional medicine, according to the science-based biomedical model, effectively "reduces illness to the operation of mechanical processes" and illness based upon subjective means is different from disease based upon objective testing (p. 4). Gadamer (1996) stresses that the responsibility of health is shared but falls greatly upon the patient. The historical moment allows for more than one answer to be correct, and this historical moment allows for alternative answers to pain other than simply taking an opioid.

Chapter Two

Crisis Communication and the Opioid Crisis

This chapter explores crisis literature and is a textual analysis of crisis literature texts. This chapter also provides an analysis of selected health crises including the shifting medical opinions on mask-wearing during the COVID-19 crisis, the shifting opinions on smoking, and the crises that ensued because of erroneous scientific recommendations. It also mentions various other health crises that encourage thought to the shifting medical rhetoric on issues. These crises were selected because these examples highlight the rhetorical shifts in the medical literature, and how the shifting rhetoric can create conflicting views in the medical community. The smoking health crisis informs how we might make sense of the opioid epidemic currently.

Theorizing Crisis Communication outlines the principles of crisis, what constitutes a crisis, and the connection between communication and crisis. Additionally, I will examine Fearn-Banks's (2016) *Crisis Communications: A Casebook Approach*. Crises shape our perceptions (Coombs and Holladay, 2009). When a situation is labeled a crisis, this is a signal for those in society to take note of the severity of a particular issue. Foundational texts, along with *The Handbook of Health Communication*, will allow me to explore the history of selected health crises in America (smoking, alcohol, and trans fats) via a scholarly lens. Exploring the question of how does rhetoric relate to the framing of the opioid crisis is addressed in this chapter because this chapter seeks to answer: What is a crisis? What theories are applicable to crisis management? What health crises have occurred in the past?

2.1 INTRODUCTION

The idea that modernity is *a risk culture* includes a preoccupation with global health crises framed as unpredictable and uncontrollable (Giddens, 2013; Pan and Ming, 2016). The news media have an essential role in giving publicity and meaning to numerous health crises of global suffering: "people around the world can perceive health crises through news coverage, given that news frames lead to various interpretations of crises" (Pan and Meng, 2016, p. 95). The news media play a dynamic role in delivering health-risk information and what health-related organizations are doing to control and combat a health crisis (Pan and Meng, 2016, p. 95). Health crises, risk management, and understanding of the diffusion of health-related information are all relevant when considering modernity and crisis communication. The media is important in creating frames around health crises.

Health crises have existed since antiquity. A crisis that once plagued many was childbirth. In ancient Rome, childbirth was a hazardous event for both mother and child, with high rates of infant and maternal mortality (Todman, 2007, p. 82). Also, in the Middle Ages, the crisis of the Bubonic Plague killed millions (Platt, 2014). In modernity, obesity, Ebola, Zika, and COVID-19 have threatened public safety. From a public health standpoint, health crises are important to control because they can quickly become unmanageable and cause human suffering and even large loss of human life. Crises receive both media coverage and scholarly attention while also attracting the attention of public health officials. For example, Cobb et al. (2010) explain the dangers of vapor cigarettes; Ebbeling, Dorota, and Pawlak (2002) seek to understand the crisis that threatens the nations' most vulnerable citizens with their research on childhood obesity; and Sutton et al. look to the HIV/AIDS crisis in their research. When the research is released to the public about a particular crisis, the researchers often reach conclusions seeking behavioral changes from the public. The behavioral changes can be as simple as avoiding vapor cigarettes or as complex as changing daily eating habits, monitoring heart rates during exercise, and counting calories.

Most recently, COVID-19 was first presented to the American public as not being a widespread threat to the United States, and in March 2020 many public health professionals were urging the public to not wear masks. The frame seemed to shift as to who needed a mask and when one should wear a mask. Early in the outbreak, the message was clear to not wear a mask; "Though health officials have warned Americans to prepare for the spread of the novel coronavirus in the U.S., people shouldn't wear face masks to prevent the spread of the infectious illness, according to the Centers for Disease Control and Prevention, the U.S. Department of Health and Human Services and the U.S. surgeon general" (Buchwald, 2020, para 1). Now, the media and public health officials are urging mask-wearing in public spaces, and mask-wearing is seen as a primary tool in defeating the virus. Hence, the media has the power to disseminate useful health information. Reaching the public with a clear message in times of a health crisis is important to improving health outcomes. In times of a health crisis, a crisis communication system should be established for the public and affected groups for uncertainty reduction, self-efficacy, and reassurance (Reynolds et al. in Pan and Meng, 2016, p. 103).

The opioid crisis has taken too many human lives and is worthy of news coverage as well as scholarly attention. "Seventy-eight people die every day in the United States from an opioid overdose," and there are long-lasting consequences associated with this crisis (Enomoto in U.S. Department of Health and Human Services & Centers for Disease Control and Prevention, 2016, p. iii). The media, doctors, pain societies, and pharmaceutical companies framed opioids as the panacea of pain management. This type of information prolonged the opioid crisis. Now the same groups are now urging people to use caution when considering opioids. Crisis communication and health communication intersect with the opioid crisis. The goal at the intersection of crisis communication and health communication involves disseminating information and changing behaviors. Doctors and patients alike need to understand the dangers of opioids and change their behavior in both prescribing and taking the drugs.

2.2 WHAT IS A CRISIS?

Individuals, organizations, and governments can trigger a crisis when acting in a way that is illegal or outside the bounds of an ethical framework established by a corporation, or simply by making a bad decision. Additionally, natural disasters, loss of power and water service for extended periods of time, or a breach in Internet security can trigger a crisis (Fearn-Banks, 2016; Sellnow and Seeger, 2013). Hearit stresses a crisis in a corporate setting is often "self-generated" and the result of "internal screw-ups" and not an external source (2006, p. 2). A crisis can be defined as "the perception of an unpredictable event that threatens important expectancies of stakeholders and can seriously impact an organization's performance and generate negative outcomes" (Coombs, 2014). Fearn-Banks (2016) describes a crisis as

> a major occurrence with a potentially negative outcome affecting the organization, company, or industry, as well as its publics, products, services, or good name. A crisis interrupts normal business transactions and can sometimes threaten the existence of the organization. The size of the organization is irrelevant. It can be a multinational corporation, a one-person business, or even an individual. (p. 2)

According to Pearson and Clair, "crises are by definition interdisciplinary events and often reach across regional, cultural, economic, and political boundaries. . . . This interdisciplinary aspect has made integration of research and practice more challenging (Pearson and Clair in Sellnow and Seeger, 2013, p. 2). The BP oil spill, Chipotle's food contamination, and the lack of federal government attention to the victims of Hurricane Katrina are all examples of crises from different economic and academic spheres: environmental, health, and governmental crises.

The magnitude of the crisis can be understood by the amount of people it reaches. Questions arise such as Is this a small-scale community issue? Or a widespread issue effecting an entire country or geographic region? The answers to these questions often provide insight into the magnitude of the crisis. Crises can occur on a small scale. For example, a single local restaurant could be serving food with high levels of *E. Coli* bacteria; the potential number of crisis victims are limited to a small customer base and geographic location. In contrast, an *E. Coli* outbreak in a national chain of restaurants affects a larger customer base.

Managing information and managing meaning are two areas of interest when learning from a crisis. Specific pieces of information such as the amount of people put at risk or the factors leading to the cause of the crisis are a part of "managing information" in the times of crisis. Coombs explains "Managing information involves the collection, analysis, and dissemination of information during a crisis" (Coombs, 2014, p. 7). A part of managing information is reviewing what was released to internal and external stakeholders, this process is often in flux as new information becomes available and reviewed in formal case studies. "Managing meaning involves the messages used in attempts to shape how people perceive the crisis or the organization in crisis" (Coombs, 2014, p. 7). Meaning arises from the formal case study when actions and behaviors are explained in context in the postcrisis phase.

Coombs (2014) explains the interpretive work of understanding and creating meaning is linked to "behavior when it seeks to influence how people interpret those actions or events" (Coombs, 2014, p. 8). In other words, once the crisis is over, people construct ideas of what happened and why and communicate the meaning to others. The crisis situation becomes retrospectively meaningful to the organization or the community that was affected. Those who study crises seek to understand how the crisis is remembered and if there are any long-lasting effects. Retrospective learning about and from a crisis occurs in the postcrisis phase.

2.3 FORMAL CASE STUDY: AN APPROACH TO CRISIS

This book in many ways serves as a case study of the opioid crisis. This text traces the precrisis, crisis, and postcrisis phase. The formal case study approach involves a thorough account of the precrisis, crisis, and postcrisis phase. "Crisis research and theory has been driven largely by crisis management practice. Initially, practitioners sought to develop frameworks and models to promote understanding and improve their practice." Over time the primary method and framework for studying a crisis is a formalized case study (Sellnow and Seeger, 2013, p. 3). Formal case study is "the systematic analysis of a case" (Coombs, 2014, p. 1). In the case study approach, "experience-based approaches eventually evolved into formal case studies." Surveys, interviews, and ethnographic research become important in the formal case study approach (Sellnow and Seeger, 2013, p. 3). Further, understanding individuals' competing narratives, both internal and external to the organization, aid in understanding the competing interests that often exist when studying crisis. For example, a company may want to limit its involvement in the crisis and construct a narrative that minimizes its role. On the other hand, community members who have been affected greatly may construct a narrative highlighting their plight.

Crisis management practice entails how one manages the public opinion. Coombs defines crisis management as "managing meaning involves the messages used in attempts to shape how people perceive the crisis or the organization in crisis" (Coombs, 2014, p. 7). Coombs and Holladay have studied how perception of a crisis is impacted with the inclusion of images while communicating about a crisis to the public. They concluded, "The inclusion of images featuring victims of a crisis could intensify attributions of crisis responsibility. As people consider the victims and sense greater danger, they could judge the organization as more responsible for the crisis" (Coombs and Holladay, 2009, p. 123). In summary, the inclusion of "real" people who have been impacted by the crisis does shape peoples' thoughts and the importance of holding those responsible for the crisis accountable. Coombs and Holladay's conclusion that including images of actual victims increases the amount of responsibility people feel an organization has to fixing the problem has been extracted from studying a myriad of formal case studies. Learning from a crisis and learning about crisis management can be accomplished by studying formal case studies. The learning phase is the fifth and final phase of a crisis in Fearn-Banks's (2016) stages of a crisis. Looking retrospectively at a crisis in the learning phase encourages strategies to prevent the situation from occurring again and provides a learning model for other organizations. The case study approach to crisis communication is a pedagogical tool of interest to those learning about theory and praxis (Coombs, 2014). Both scholars and public relations professionals employ the formal case study approach to learn.

2.4 THREE-STAGE MODEL

Sellnow and Seeger (2013) suggest that most crises can be evaluated in three main parts. The three-stage model for studying a crisis breaks the crisis into three parts: precrisis, crisis, and postcrisis. This model has been adopted widely by organizational crisis theorists and communication scholars and is probably the most widely used framework due, in part, to its simplicity (Sellnow and Seeger, 2013, p. 31). These phases become applicable when thinking about how the opioid crisis evolved. During precrisis, an emerging threat or some type of uncertainty develops and interacts with other aspects of a corporate structure, organization, or system. The looming uncertainty is described as

> an incubation or gestation process where the magnitude of a threat grows and creates dynamic non-linear interactions. Often, this incubation involves a risk judged by managers as minor, interacting in a non-linear and disproportional way with other factors. In some cases, threats converge or connect and interact with other deficiencies or fallacious assumptions about risk. (Sellnow and Seeger, 2013, p. 31)

From Seeger and Sellnow's description of the precrisis stage, there are clear signs of an impending crisis, which individuals closest to the organization may be able to recognize.

The crisis phase begins with a trigger event and a general recognition that a crisis has indeed occurred. A trigger event can be a "sudden occurrence that signals a severe disruption of the system and onset of harm or the potential for harm," such as a fire, explosion, or flood (Sellnow and Seeger, 2013, p. 31). In other cases, a trigger event may be "subtle" and involve a realization that a crisis is developing as information is accumulated and interpreted. The recognition of a crisis is "often accompanied by extreme emotional arousal, stress, fear, anger, shock, general disbelief and sometimes denial" (Sellnow and Seeger, 2013, p. 31). The crisis serves as a rhetorical interruption severing the mundane everyday chain of events and replacing it with uncertainty.

The postcrisis begins when the "harm, drama, confusion and uncertainty of the crisis dissipate and some sense of order is re-established" (Sellnow and Seeger, 2013, p. 32). The postcrisis, referred to as the learning stage by Fearn-Banks (2016). The postcrisis phase "is a time of intense investigation and analysis that includes efforts to create plausible explanations of what went wrong; why, how, who is to blame; and what should be done to prevent future crises" (Sellnow and Seeger, 2013, p. 32). Isolating and reviewing the trigger event is seen as important for preventing future crises.

In addition to the case study approach, learning from a formal case study should also take into consideration ideas of culture and community. Communal norms are often violated in a crisis situation. Sellnow and Seeger (2013) note, "Crises involve a radical departure from the status quo and a violation of general assumptions and expectations, disrupting the 'normal' and limiting the ability to anticipate and predict. The severe violation of expectations is usually a source of uncertainty, psychological discomfort and stress" (p. 6). Crises disrupt everyday existence and serve as a rhetorical interruption by disturbing the flow of everyday life. During a crisis, life departs from routine and becomes unpredictable, and "significant threats to such high priority goals as life, property, security, health and psychological stability are often associated with crises" (Sellnow and Seeger, 2013, p. 7).

The work of Karl Weick is relevant when examining a culture of uncertainty after a crisis. Weick explains that, as life becomes more unpredictable, "equivocality" is heightened. Weick wrote *The Social Psychology of Organizing* in 1979 and both coined and defined the term "equivocality." Equivocality is the extent to which data are unclear and suggest two or more interpretations about the environment; additionally, the receiver is left with uncertainty (Weick, 1979, p. 180). Weick argues that successful organizations reduce equivocality through sharing observations and discussion until a common grammar and course of action can be reached (Weick, 1979, p. 180–183). In other words, communicating about a plan using shared *grammar* can reduce uncertainty in the organization. The culture of an organization can be changed forever in the postcrisis phase.

2.5 INTERSECTION OF CRISIS COMMUNICATION AND HEALTH COMMUNICATION

This project is situated at the intersection of health communication and crisis communication. The manner in which the medical community communicates to the public in times of crisis is important in taking preventive measures and saving lives. Mass media journalists often attempt to "sensationalize news stories to stir up panic and prosecute government entities regardless of their effort," but effective communication campaigns launched from government entities tend to focus on behavioral changes and not on personal narratives or ad hominem attacks (Pan and Meng, 2016, p. 105). Effective communication campaigns are often launched from a federal health agency such as the CDC and the Food and Drug Administration (FDA). For a campaign to be successful, it must reach its target audience. The following is one method for assuring that the target audience receives the campaign's message: CDC licenses the annual American Healthstyles survey for audience analysis (U.S. Department of Health and Human Services & Centers for Disease Control and Prevention, 2017), and the Health Information National Trends Survey (HINTS) provides research on a representative U.S. sample of adults specific to cancer and includes information on channel usage, risk perceptions, and use of information as well as demographic information (National Cancer Institute 2009 in Thompson et al., 2011, p. 196). These research campaigns provide information for communication professionals to segment their audiences across several variables so that messages can be tailored to the appropriate audience.

Much data from the American Healthstyles survey have yielded anti-smoking campaigns, and this information may help to inform future campaigns constructed to combat the opioid crisis. The smoking crisis informs the opioid crisis as it, too, is located at the intersection of health communication and crisis communication. The smoking crisis and the opioid crisis both benefit when the physician or health-sponsored agency communicates a clear health-related message (i.e., do not smoke as it causes cancer or do not take opioids as they lead to addiction). Research has demonstrated that health communication campaigns can effectively address important global public health issues such as HIV/AIDS prevention and smoking cessation (Allen et al., 2015; Olawepo et al., 2019). Furlan et al. (2018) conducted a systematic review of the effectiveness of various strategies to reduce opioid use disorder and opioid overdose deaths and, based on limited evidence from five studies, found communication campaigns to be one of the most promising strategies. Furlan et al. (2018) concluded the content of the communication campaigns matters and campaigns should include education, clinical practice changes, naloxone distribution, regulations, collaborations, public health, and opioid substitution treatments.

The remaining parts of this chapter are dedicated to drawing connections between the opioid crisis and the smoking crisis, focusing on the importance of empowering patients in their health care decisions, and recognizing that paradigmatic shifts in the medical community can cause catastrophes for some patients.

2.5.1 A Scholarly Lens to the Smoking Crisis in America

Just like the opioid crisis, the smoking crisis in America can be traced to the endorsement of cigarette smoking by medical professionals and to advertising of "the health benefits" of cigarettes. Allan Brandt, a professor of History of Medicine and of the History of Science at Harvard, has written several books, including *The Cigarette Century: The Rise, Fall, and Deadly Persistence of the Product That Defined America* in 2007, which was a finalist for the Pulitzer Prize. In this book, Brandt traces the history of cigarettes and the public health crisis caused by cigarette smoking. Cigarette smoking is the "primary causal factor for at least 30% of all cancer deaths, for nearly 80% of deaths from chronic obstructive pulmonary disease, and for early cardiovascular disease and deaths" (Centers for Disease Control and Prevention, 2008, p. 1226). In addition, exposure to secondhand smoke increases risks for cancer, chronic obstructive pulmonary disease, and cardiovascular disease, as well as irritation of the throat, lungs, and eyes.

Beginning in 1946, "a major new advertising campaign for Camel cigarettes centered on the memorable slogan 'More Doctors Smoke Camels Than Any Other Cigarette'" (Brandt, 2007, p. 105). This advertising campaign suggested that the Camel brand had consulted every doctor in private practice in the United States and that they had overwhelmingly recommended Camel cigarettes. The American Medical Association (AMA) convention of 1947 was held in Atlantic City, and doctors stood in long lines to receive free cigarettes. Additionally, "the Philip Morris display at the convention explained the advantages of diethylene glycol as a hygroscopic agent, insisting it was the healthiest cigarette" (Brandt, 2007, p. 105). While the advertising campaigns were reaching the public in the 1940s and shaping their opinion that cigarettes had health benefits, scientists in both the United States and the United Kingdom were exploring the risks of smoking and adverse health effects.

Chesterfield cigarettes—which were advertised as "Chesterfield Best for You!"—attempted to convince the public that Chesterfield was the healthier alternative to other cigarettes. Chesterfield advertisements coincided with news of the studies that appeared beginning in 1950 linking smoking to lung cancer (Brandt, 2007, p. 394–395). Even broadcaster "Arthur Godfrey, who regularly pitched Chesterfields on his televised variety show, promised 'No adverse effects to the nose, throat, and sinuses from smoking Chesterfield.' Godfrey survived the removal of a lung tumor in 1959 but succumbed to emphysema in 1983" (Brandt, 2007, p. 394). It was clear that Chesterfield cigarettes were not the "Best for You" as evidence began to appear linking the cigarettes and disease.

The crisis of tobacco usage was leading to the epidemic rates of lung cancer. In the 1950s, statisticians E. Cuyler Hammond and Daniel Horn simultaneously conducted a prospective study under the auspices of the American Cancer Society; their findings concurred with the numerous studies from the United Kingdom that linked cigarettes to lung cancer. Hammond states:

> We are concerned here with a restricted set of conditions—human populations where death from infectious and parasitic diseases is uncommon and where violence and accidents account for a relatively small proportion of all deaths. It is only in such populations that a remarkable degree of association has been found between death rates and amount of cigarette smoking. (Brandt, 2007, p. 146)

Health communication was of vital importance during the next five decades. Health communication literature needed to change the mindset of doctors and the public even though, approximately four years before Hammond's study was released, doctors were lining up at the AMA conference for free cigarettes. The health communication literature needed most at this time addressed changing the behaviors and mindsets of physicians and patients alike.

In 1957, the first official statement from the U.S. Public Health Service was released, implicating that smoking as a causative factor in lung cancer had been established to a high degree of scientific certainty, although it was not until later that the 1964 Surgeon General Advisory Committee report was able to shift public opinion (Cummings and Proctor, 2014, p. 33). The 1964 Surgeon General's report received much media attention, especially the section stating, "The risk of developing lung cancer increases with duration of smoking and the number of cigarettes smoked per day, and is diminished by discontinuing smoking" (1). Public perception also shifted in 1966 when the first cautionary label appeared on cigarette packs, advising that cigarette smoking "may be hazardous to your health" (Cummings and Proctor, 2014, p. 34). People became fearful and began to change their behaviors.

These health communication campaigns were successful in that there was a decline in "adult per-capita cigarette consumption" in 1964 as the dangers of smoking became better known and regulation increased on the sale and advertising of tobacco (Cummings and Proctor, 2014, p. 34). In 1967, anti-smoking advertisements began to air on television as part of a Federal Communications Commission Fairness Doctrine ruling that required broadcasters to run an anti-smoking advertisement for every cigarette advertisement aired. The ratio of 1:1 was not strictly followed, but smoking rates declined (Cummings and Proctor, 2014, p. 33–34). Cigarette advertisements were banned from television and radio in 1971, and, about this time, public perception of smoking began to shift, making smoking less socially acceptable.

However, more than thirty years after the data was publicly released that linked smoking and cancer, some Americans remain unsure: "In 2001 Gallup re-asked this same question and found 71% of Americans naming smoking as a major cause of cancer, with 11% saying it was a minor cause and 16% unsure" (Cummings and Proctor, 2014, p. 33). Despite the overwhelming evidence that cigarettes kill, "none of these companies has ever admitted that millions of people have died as a result of smoking their products or that addiction to nicotine can cause death" (Cummings and Proctor, 2014, p. 36). But overall, health communication campaigns disseminated the information linking cigarette smoking and cancer and have successfully changed consumer behaviors and physician recommendations concerning cigarettes.

2.6 DISCUSSION AND CONNECTIONS TO THE CURRENT OPIOID CRISIS

According to Brandt, cigarette smoking was once endorsed by the medical community as a treatment for several health ailments, and, over the course of five decades, health communication literature helped shape public opinion against the usage of tobacco products. Opioids, too, were once endorsed indiscriminately as the first line of treatment for many nonspecific acute and chronic forms of pain before exhausting less harmful alternatives. Lopez (2017) gives the following account:

Back in the 1990s, doctors were persuaded to treat pain as a serious medical issue. There's a good reason for that: About 100 million U.S. adults suffer from chronic pain, according to a 2011 report from the Institute of Medicine. Pharmaceutical companies took advantage of this concern. Through a big marketing campaign, they got doctors to prescribe products like OxyContin and Percocet in droves—even though the evidence for opioids treating long-term, chronic pain is very weak (despite their effectiveness for short-term, acute pain), while the evidence that opioids cause harm in the long term is very strong.

Doctors succumbed to the marketing campaigns and prescribed opioids; once people began using the opioids, they quickly became addicted or physically dependent on these medicines.

Legislatures are now suing the opioid manufacturers and forcing opioid manufacturers to take responsibility. One lawsuit filer is the State of Ohio, which is "accusing several drug companies of conducting marketing campaigns that misled doctors and patients about the dangers of addiction and overdose" (Perez-Pena, 2017). The tobacco industry was once similarly sued by states; the resulting Master Settlement Agreement required the four largest tobacco companies to stop marketing to children and to pay the states money to care for those adversely affected by cigarettes.

Opinions in the scientific community have shifted significantly since the early 1900s, and there is widespread agreement that smoking negatively impacts health. The overarching scientific community's thoughts are still undecided on opioids; though widespread agreement exists that we are among epidemic proportions of opioid-related deaths due to overuse. As complexity theory states, there are several variables that need to be addressed when considering the opioid crisis; the patient community, the medical community, the pharmaceutical industry, and on an institutional level, the American Medical Association, the Drug Enforcement Agency, and the Food and Drug Administration are all stakeholders that need to be included and participate in ending the crisis. All of these groups recognize the crisis but have not yet communicated a plan to the public on plans of ending the crisis. The next chapter will explore the rhetorical nature of science and how paradigms shift.

2.7 HEALTH CRISES

Crises affecting people's health and well-being are often studied at the intersection of two disciplinary studies; crisis communication and health communication. For over twenty years, Renata Schiavo, Ph.D., M.A., has worked at the interface of health equity, health systems, community health, community and patient engagement, strategy design, international development, social marketing, risk communication, and cross-cultural communication for behavioral, social, and organizational change to improve health and social outcomes among different populations. Schiavo's work explores the importance of effective health communication in times of crisis and outbreaks.

Schiavo explains an intersection of health communication and crisis communication with the classic example of the childhood illnesses and communal outbreaks of polio, measles, mumps, rubella, and whooping cough. In this example, immunization rates increased as health communication literature became more widely disseminated during outbreaks. Schiavo writes, however, that

> for most other health-related issues and interventions, changing public and professional minds and enabling parents to immunize their healthy children have required a worldwide multidisciplinary effort. Health communication has played a fundamental role in this success story since the introduction of the first childhood vaccine. (Schiavo, 2013, p. xxiii)

Health communication literature in times of a health crisis must address both the behavior and mentality of the physician, the community, and the patients. Changing behavior in a time of a crisis is often necessary, though more difficult.

Another element relevant to the health communication literature is health literacy. Health literacy is defined as "[the] degree to which individuals have the capacity to obtain, process, and understand basic health information and services needed to make appropriate health decisions" (Kutner et al., 2006, p. iii). Health literacy traditionally focused on the doctor-patient relationship. In doing so, the focus of health literacy was how to improve the explanation of medical terms and choices in clinical visits. More relevant than the doctor-patient relations are the health decisions every day that individuals make, and not all situations allow for thorough explanations of the health risks at hand. Particularly in crises that create health risks, like food-borne outbreaks, individuals with limited health literacy are at even more of a disadvantage (Roberts and Veil, 2015, p. 123). Adults living below the poverty line had lower average health literacy than adults living above the poverty threshold (Kutner et al., 2006, p. v). Efforts to include still imagery and video in online news stories help to address meeting the needs of all levels of health literacy; below basic, basic, and proficient.

Health literacy requires an individual to possess at least the basic skills of being able to read as well as listen and to possess the ability to make decisions while being analytical. An individual must be, "visually literate (able to understand graphs or other visual information), computer literate (able to operate a computer), information literate (able to obtain and apply relevant information), and numerically or computationally literate (able to calculate or reason numerically)," and be able to apply all these skills to personal health (Roberts and Veil, 2015, p. 125). Television is the primary means used to reach the public in a health crisis situation (Roberts and Veil, 2015, p. 125). Attaining proficiency in health literacy leads to better health outcomes and a greater sense of empowerment over one's health.

2.8 PATIENT-PROVIDER COMMUNICATION AND AGENCY

Barbara M. Korsch, M.D., a pioneer in the field of health communication, identified issues with the way the medical community was communicating with the patient community. Korsch (2011) relies on her clinical and research experience to attest to the importance of the study of health communication. She writes,

> When clinicians and scientists first called attention to the need for improvement of this aspect (health communication) of health care delivery, there had been little scientific investigation or explicit attention to the subject. It was then considered part of the "art of medicine," which came naturally or not, depending on the personality of the professionals involved. The doctor-patient relationship was sacred and could not be challenged and hence could neither be studied nor taught. (p. i)

Attention to the field of health communication and the importance of it has flourished because of an empowered patient community; this empowered community came forward with honest assessments of how their doctors treated them and what they were lacking in their treatment (Korsch, 2011). Epstein and Street (2011) note philosophically, patient-centered care as an approach to care is the right thing to do. Behaviors associated with patient-centered care, such as respecting patients' preferences, should be justified on moral grounds alone, independent of their relationship to health outcomes. Korsch (2011) notes that the process required "a more vocal, self-confident patient community" aware of their rights, but there still is much work to be done. One part of health communication is the doctor-patient relationship, but more important is the way the medical community communicates with the patient community. Street, Makoul, Arora, and Epstein (2009) report patients have overall better health outcomes when there is open patient-clinician communication that incorporates trust and shared decision-making. Epstein and Street (2011) highlight an important distinction; patient-centered care does not mean writing prescriptions just because the patient requests them; inappropriate prescribing is not patient-centered care.

Several distinct disciplinary areas of study guide the development of health communication. Sociology, psychology, and communication are fundamental in understanding the field of health communication. According to Parrot and Krueter, "the journal *Sociology of Health and Illness* was first published in 1978; the journal *Health Psychology* was first published in 1981; and the journal *Health Communication* was first published in 1989" (quoted in Thompson et al., 2011, p. iii). Research published in the aforementioned journals is indicative of the "biopsychosocial" approach to health and illness. By exploring roles of biological, psychological, and social factors, a biopsychosocial approach is a type of holistic approach to health that acknowledges the body-mind connection and a connection between individual and community health. Health communication seeks to transcend disciplinary boundaries. "Integrative models that include medical and epidemiological approaches in concert with behavioral science approaches" lead to innovations and insights that go beyond one discipline's theories and systems (Parrot and Kreuter in Thompson et al., 2011, p. 5).

For example, two disciplines—health communication and mass communication—have transcended boundaries to make discoveries for improving public outreach and public health. Parrot and Krueter suggest that *The Journal of Health and Mass Communication*'s appearance in 2009 highlights "the growing emphasis on understanding the role of mass communication, an example of a subdiscipline within communication which makes significant contributions to health communication" (Thompson et al., 2015, p. iii). Mass communication involves disseminating information to the public via radio, television, print media, and the Internet. News media play an essential role in giving publicity and meaning to several health crises involving global suffering (Pan and Meng, 2016, p. 95). People around the world perceive health crises through news coverage, given that news frames lead to various interpretations of health crises by highlighting and including certain aspects while refusing to include others (Dutton and Ashford in Pan and Meng, 2016,

p. 95). Fairhust and Sarr's (1996) work on framing, which is analyzed in later chapters of this project, seeks to understand how health professionals employed certain frames to patients regarding risks of taking prescription opioids, and how pain societies framed prescribing of opioids to physicians.

Advertising of medicines and health products is an example of both health communication and mass-media communication. The marketing of over-the-counter (OTC) drugs increased dramatically in 1972 as many drugs became available without a prescription. Advertising is intended to shape consumer behavior to purchase; in fact, "the Nonprescription Drug Marketing Association (NDMA), has claimed Americans rely on advertising as a major OTC drug information source" (Thompson et al., 2011, p. 269). Economic and financial implications cannot be overlooked when considering drug advertising. "OTC drug advertising also plays a role in the larger American economy. . . . Market competition and advertising's economic contributions are closely associated" (Thompson et al., 2011, p. 270). Ethical questions arise when considering advertising medications. Some questions involve if the consumer is in the position to make the appropriate choice and if the consumer is being persuaded to try an unneeded medication. Exploring how medicines and health products have been advertised in the past may provide a more nuanced view of the complex questions that arise when studying the connection between these products and public health.

Chapter Three

The Rhetoric of the Opioid Crisis and the Relationship between Rhetoric and Framing Theory

3.1 INTRODUCTION

This chapter seeks to answer how the rhetorical nature of science impacts the terms "addiction" and "addict," especially related to the opioid crisis; how the rhetorical nature of science impacts how doctors treat their patients; and how to define a moral failing or a brain-based disease. This chapter argues science is rhetorical and rhetoric is the basis of having people buy in and believe or not believe in an idea. Rhetoric and persuasion are the basis of encouraging behavioral change of another. Aristotle explained rhetoric boils down to persuasion, and the history of rhetoric is explored in this chapter (2011b).

The rhetoric of the opioid crisis has had a profound role in shaping society's interpretation of and reaction to the crisis. Many people expect drugs to solve pain problems, and they marginalize the role of self-driven, nonopioid solutions in treating pain (Gourlay et al., 2005, p. 112–117; Catan et al., 2013, p. 123–128). This mindset could be attributed to the Enlightenment, which created a false sense of hope that science could fix all problems (Arnett, 2012, p. 18–20). This rhetoric of pain treatment has similarly impacted the physician-patient relationship. Patients expect a quick-fix medication prescription rather than options, such as active exercise and cognitive behavioral therapy that require more patient commitment; such options, however, have been shown to have more success and fewer adverse effects in treating chronic pain (Rainville et al., 2004, p. 106). Giddens (2013) explains the idea of a scientific outlook in modernity often "excludes questions of ethics or morality," and the lack of ethical actions by pharmaceutical companies, doctors, and pain societies contributed to opioid abuse (Giddens, 2013, p. 8; Lembke, 2016, p. 30–115). Interdisciplinary programs that include cognitive behavior therapy are often denied by insurers due to the cost, hence focusing the attention on profits and not on the welfare of the insured (Meldrum, 2016, p. 1365).

Rhetoric's relationship to science has long been explored. Plato, Aristotle, and Cicero in antiquity understood the power of rhetoric as each contributed to rhetorical theory and how information is disseminated to the public (Gross and Keith, 1997, p. 26–29). The relationship between science and "Truth" was illuminated during the height of the Enlightenment in the eighteenth century, but, in this postmodern modern moment, "we live in a time when disillusionment more often than the hope of Truth promised by the Enlightenment defines us" (Arnett, Fritz, and Bell, 2008, p. 2). The Enlightenment brought with it the hope that *rational thought and reason* could liberate a person from the past (Arnett, 2012, p. 19). In other words, the Enlightenment brought false hope that scientific rationality could solve most problems.

This mode of thinking has created an overreliance on pharmacology and the medical community to treat pain (Catt, 2012, p. 81–100). In postmodern America, when people experience pain, they want the pain to disappear, and they too often turn to pharmacological options for relief of all types of pain (Catt, 2012, p. 81–100). However, after taking the opioids, their pain is still there. Opioids have tremendous externalities associated with them, the most serious being addiction.

This chapter also explores the unresolved, challenging, and politically volatile question of addiction being either a moral failing or a brain-based disease, and how society's views on the nature of addiction shape the rhetoric of chronic pain treatment both in the doctor's office and in society at large (U.S. Department of Health and Human Services & Centers for Disease Control and Prevention, 2016, p. v). To explain the rhetorical nature of science, Thomas Kuhn's (1970) *The Structure of Scientific Revolutions* defines a paradigm: a set of assumptions that shape the way one sees the world. A paradigm shift occurs when those assumptions are challenged. Rhetoric is the force that persuasively shifts the paradigm. In regard to the opioid crisis, Surgeon General Murthy (2016) calls for a paradigm shift from seeing addiction as a moral failing to a disease when he writes,

> We need to invest more in expanding the scientific evidence base for prevention, treatment, and recovery. We also need a cultural shift in how we think about addiction. For far too long, too many in our country have viewed addiction as a moral failing. This unfortunate stigma has created an added burden of shame that has made people with substance use disorders less likely to come forward and seek help. It has also made it more challenging to marshal the necessary

> investments in prevention and treatment. We must help everyone see that addiction is not a character flaw—it is a chronic illness that we must approach with the same skill and compassion with which we approach heart disease, diabetes, and cancer. (p. v)

This chapter focuses defining rhetoric and generating a rhetorical understanding of the concepts of an addict, addiction, and drug abuse, as well as the paradigm shifts that have occurred. I will explore the foundational article in Goffman's *Framing Theory, Frame Analysis: An Essay on the Organization of Experience*, (1974) and further application of framing from Fairhurst and Sarr's theory. Finally, I will look at the framing of addiction—a moral failing or an illness (Holton, 2016, p. 300–303; Pickard, 2016, p. 277)?

3.2 WHAT IS RHETORIC?

The study of rhetoric has a rich historic tradition with roots in antiquity (Pernot, 2005, p. ix). Plato's fourth-century dialogue *Gorgias* is one of the earliest works that uses the term "rhetoric" (Pernot, 2005, p. 15). *Gorgias* opens with Gorgias concluding a speech to the community, after which Socrates asks, "What art does he profess?" (Plato, 380 BCE, p. 1). Gorgias replies that his is the art of rhetoric. Gorgias explains a powerful rhetorician can have "the trainer as his slave" or "the physician as his slave" (Plato, 380 BCE, p. 1). The character Socrates soon concludes that Gorgias is practicing a "false art" akin to "cosmetics" or "cookery" (Plato, 380 BCE, p. 2). True arts, according to Plato, such as medicine or gymnastics, bring people closer to some truth. Rhetoric for Plato was a "knack," a "false art," and Plato denounces rhetoric throughout the dialogue, especially Sophist rhetoric (Pernot, 2005, p. 48). Sophist rhetoric sought to construct any plausible truth with disregard for the actual truth.

Cicero (106–43 BCE), a great Roman orator and rhetorical theorist, responds to Plato's *Gorgias* in his dialogue *De Oratore* (Vasaly, 1996, p. 26). *De Oratore* is a mature work on rhetoric completed when Cicero was older and more experienced and offers a retort to Plato's criticisms of the art of rhetoric (Vasaly, 1996, p. 26–28). *De Oratore* is composed as a dialogue but does not resemble Plato's argumentative dialogues; rather, the participants—Crassus, Antonius, Rufus, and Cotta—cooperate to contribute insights about rhetoric (Vasaly, 1996, p. 26–31). Cicero stresses the need for a union between tongue and brain, meaning that eloquence and wisdom must both be present and that "empty" rhetoric, or eloquence without wisdom or content, does not help the community. Cicero writes, "In the orator we must demand the subtlety of a logician, the thoughts of the philosopher, a diction almost poetic, a lawyer's memory, a tragedian's voice, and the bearing of the most consummate actor" (2019, p. 1.28.128). An "ideal" orator is rare but has the skills of eloquence and wisdom. In addition, Cicero emphasizes the role of rhetoric in shaping ordinary citizens, the "res publica." Cicero explains, "Whereas in all other arts that is most excellent which is farthest removed from the understanding and mental capacity of the untrained, in oratory the very cardinal sin is to depart from the language of everyday life, and the usage approved by the sense of the community sensus" (Cicero, 2019, p. 1.3.12). To Cicero, wisdom and eloquence provide meaning, and using the language of the people and speaking in clear everyday terminology allows a connection between speaker and audience to emerge.

Plato's student Aristotle was a Greek philosopher who studied a wide range of topics including biology, zoology, metaphysics, and rhetoric. Aristotle wrote *Rhetoric and Poetics* in approximately 333 BCE. Aristotle's *Rhetoric* provides many useful definitions and categories in this research. Aristotle writes in book I that "rhetoric is the counterpart of dialectic" and that the "argumentative modes of persuasion are the essence of the art of rhetoric" (333 BCE, p. 19). Aristotle (333 BCE) defines rhetoric as "the faculty of observing in any given case the available means of persuasion" (24). In short, the purpose of rhetoric is to formulate arguments that persuade the audience to adopt the speaker's intended message.

Artistic proofs are the available means of persuasion: ethos, pathos, and logos. Ethos refers to the ethical constitution of the speaker and relies on the ethical makeup of one's character to convince. Pathos relies on the speaker's ability to "stir the emotions" of the listeners. Logos refers to the logical organization of arguments; it is the speaker's ability to list "facts" or organize talking points to "prove" a truth or apparent truth (Aristotle, 2011b, p. 24–25). In addition, Aristotle explains that "the enthymeme is the substance of rhetorical persuasion" and the "orator's demonstration of persuasion is the enthymeme" (2011b, p. 20). An enthymeme is a truncated syllogism. A formal syllogism requires the audience to draw logical conclusions about the information provided.

In addition to artistic proofs and the power of the enthymeme, Aristotle describes categories or "divisions" of rhetoric in *Rhetoric and Poetics*. Forensic rhetoric is also called "judicial" as this is the rhetoric of the courts. Forensic or judicial rhetoric is focused on past actions and is concerned with guilt or innocence (Aristotle, 2011b, p. 32). Ceremonial rhetoric, also called "epideictic," is concerned with praising or blaming and is associated with a present-time orientation. "Deliberative" or political rhetoric is focused on the future and involves a politician asking for some type of future action, usually a vote for or against a certain bill or law. Aristotle assigns each category of rhetoric its own means and ends (2011b, p. 32). The categorization of rhetoric is helpful when studying persuasive messages encouraging behavioral changes. Ceremonial rhetoric is akin to a commercial praising a product and encouraging consumption. Also, deliberative rhetoric is focused on some future action that you want someone to do or not do at a future time. The historical roots of rhetoric are largely planted in persuasion, specifically in shaping public opinion (Herrick, 2001, p. 1–20; Aristotle, 2011b, p. 1–18). The connection between rhetoric and science is worthy of investigation because rhetoric is still responsible for conveying scientific developments to the res publica.

3.3 RHETORIC AND SCIENCE

Beginning in the seventeenth century, René Descartes and Giambattista Vico debated the rule of rhetoric and its relationship to science. In *Discourse on Method,* Descartes denigrates rhetoric and emphasizes mathematics and mathematical proofs as a way to bring knowledge into the world. Descartes "[finds] the rhetorical tradition dating from antiquity irrelevant to his project" (Carr, 2009, p. ix). Vico (1990), however, criticizes Descartes as Vico argues that rhetoric is the basis for knowledge and that science is based on argument and conviction (Bizzell and Herzberg, 2001, p. 862). In *On the Study Methods of Our Time,* Vico defends the ancients' rhetorical tradition. Vico argues, "they [the Ancients] devoted all their activity to certain arts which we almost totally neglect" (p. 5). The arts of poetry and rhetoric are important to Vico because he sees rhetoric as a way to bring order into the world. Vico conceptualizes rhetoric as primarily "concerned with the education and fostering of leaders with good character and a strong commitment to the public good. [Vico's] rhetorical theory thus represents a revival of Ciceronian ideals in which rhetoric is the framework for a good society" (Hartelius, 2012, p. 155).

For Vico, "the problems that concern human beings . . . are the ones that urge themselves upon us in the construction of the human world" (Grassi, 2000, p. 6). Vico seeks to "humanize" nature by emphasizing myth, storytelling, arts, music, and poetry (Grassi, 2000, p. 6). These products of fantasy and imagination are vital to the sciences, according to Vico, because they allow people to think beyond what is directly in front of them. Vico writes, "Fantasy collects from the senses and connects and enlarges to exaggeration the sensory effects of the natural appearances and makes luminous images from them, in order to suddenly blind the mind with lightning bolts and thereby to conjure up human passions in the ringing and thunder of this astonishment" (Grassi, 2000, p. 7). Herrick (2001), a scholar of rhetoric writes, "Science's sterile method and reverence for individual reason threatened to undermine the sensus communis—common beliefs, values, and communal judgment that allowed great societies to flourish"; Vico uses rhetoric and science synergistically to combat the sterility (p. 170). Based on a belief that rhetoric and a rich humanities education could cultivate senus communis, "Vico argue[s] that rhetoric, not logic, provide[s] a reliable foundation for humane culture, and that what [Vico] term[s] poetic speech encourage[s] civilized behavior" (Herrick, 2001, p. 170). The theme of unification of wisdom and eloquence is evident in Vico's work.

Communal judgment is pertinent to understanding the opioid crisis. Decisions made during the course of everyday life are guided by prudence. "Decisions in public life were not based on certainties but on weighing options guided by prudence (prudentia) or practical judgment based on probabilities. Such decision-making wisdom (sapientia) was assisted by the eloquence (eloquentia) of trained orators" (Herrick, 2001, p. 171). Cicero's "ideal orator" influences Vico's ideas about bringing scientific wisdom to the "res publica," Cicero, too, is fully aware of the need for "ingenium" imagination and fantasy to imagine what is not yet known or seen (Crusius in Grassi, 2000, p. xv). Vico's vision for rhetoric can influence communal judgment by providing a way to invent and share new ideas in a logical way, bringing a union of wisdom and eloquence (Grassi, 2000, p. 41–44). Vico's "pedagogy posits as principal students' capacity for, and exercise in, invention" (Hartelius, 2012, p. 171); imagination, fantasy, and the capacity to think beyond the concrete world drives much scientific exploration (Verene, 1981, p. 34).

Like Vico, Thomas Kuhn also values the role of rhetoric in science. Kuhn, a physicist and a University of California professor of the history of science, details the relationship between rhetoric and science in *The Structure of Scientific Revolutions* (Hairston, 1982, p. 76). Kuhn writes that scientific knowledge can best be explained through a "paradigm" and paradigm shifts (Kuhn, 1970, p. 43–53). Kuhn explains that much of science is based in "normal science" and that normal science is based in relatively stable times of agreement. In Kuhn's work, "normal science" refers to "research firmly based upon one or more past scientific achievements, achievements that some particular scientific community acknowledges for a time as supplying the foundation for its further practice" (Kuhn, 1970, p. 10). The scientific community generally accepts normal science and its paradigms. One paradigm of normal science is a "theory must seem better than its competitors, but it need not, and in fact never does, explain all the facts with which it can be confronted" (Kuhn, 1970, p. 17–18). Scientists develop a new paradigm, as "their achievement was sufficiently unprecedented to attract an enduring group of adherents away from competing modes of scientific activity Simultaneously, it was sufficiently open-ended to leave all sorts of problems for the redefined group of practitioners to resolve" (Kuhn, 1970, p. 10). According to Kuhn, science is not linear, and the way we learn about science is not a straight line where one scientific development leads to the next. Rather, normal science enters a paradigm shift when people become dissatisfied with the existing paradigm, and a new paradigm emerges with a different way of viewing the world.

A paradigm is a rhetorically constructed collection of facts. It is a generally accepted view of facts that explain some phenomenon. When this paradigm is no longer considered sufficient, the paradigm shifts, and a new paradigm emerges (Kuhn, 1970, p. 118–120). When a paradigm shift occurs, the scientific community abandons the old paradigm and begins to move to the new paradigm to investigate any questions that may exist. When the new paradigm emerges, it is "incommensurable" or no longer compatible with the current paradigm. The new paradigm becomes "an object for further articulation and specification under new and stringent conditions" (Kuhn, 1970, p. 23). A new paradigm emerges because the new facts in the new paradigm do a better job at explaining the world: "Adherents to a new paradigm adopt an altered Weltunanschauung, prescribing a new way of observing, reflecting on, and describing the world" (Koschmann, 1996, p. 1). Paradigm shifts are rhetorical because they are largely trying to persuade people to abandon old modes of thinking. Kuhn explains that these shifts are not "neutral" nor can "be made a step at a time, forced by logic and neutral experience. Like the gestalt switch, it must occur all at once (though not necessarily in an instant) or not at all" (1996, p. 150). Times of revolutionary paradigm shifts present immense challenges as "the transfer of allegiance from paradigm to paradigm is a conversion experience that cannot be forced" (Kuhn, 1970, p. 151). Kuhn understands some scientists are unwilling to accept new paradigms. This resistance is not only due to being "stubborn" but also often comes from those "whose productive careers have committed them to an older tradition of normal science" (Kuhn, 1970, p. 151); their resistance is an expected part of human nature.

Kuhn believes, however, that it is less important to change individual scientists than to change scientific communities for a paradigm shift to succeed. Kuhn concludes the best way to encourage a shift is to answer questions the old paradigm cannot. Kuhn (1970) writes, "Probably the single most prevalent claim advanced by the proponents of a new paradigm is that they can solve the problems that have led the old one to a crisis" (p. 153). Paradigm shifts result in scientific revolutions.

In the past decade, a new paradigm has been constructed that stresses opioid therapy is not appropriate for chronic pain and conservative opioid therapy is safer than liberal prescribing. In the 1990s, efforts to improve treatment of pain using opioids failed to take into account opioids' addictiveness and lack of documented effectiveness in the treatment of chronic pain, and the old paradigm of liberal opioid prescribing was questioned by many in the scientific community (Frieden and Houry, 2016). On March 15, 2016, the CDC released new guidelines encouraging nonopioid therapy for the treatment of chronic pain (Centers for Disease Control and Prevention, 2016). The shift wasn't adopted by all physicians and there is and was resistance to the CDC guidelines (Renthal, 2016; Rose, 2018).

Kuhn recognizes not everyone will shift their views without resistance. Sometimes, Kuhn explains, it takes the death of an entire generation of scientists before the new paradigm is fully recognized. Some people try to make ad hoc changes to existing paradigms, or they ignore contradictions to resist the shifting paradigms (Hairston, 1982, p. 76). Those who cling to old paradigms often lose influence in their field; when their work is ignored, the shift is complete, and what was once revolutionary becomes conventional (Hairston, 1982, p. 77).

Alan Gross, a scholar of rhetoric of science, explores the link between rhetoric and science. Gross explains to readers science policy involves issues that "fall readily within the traditional concerns of those trained in rhetorical analysis" (Gross, 2006, p. 4). Understanding science hermeneutically as an epistemology allows science to be viewed as a source of "epistemology based on understanding"; hence, paradigms shift as understandings of scientific episteme change (Gross, 1990, p. 92). Gross's work brings to the forefront that scientists must "convince themselves and others that the assertions they make are an integral part of the privileged activity to which they are aligned" (Gross, 1990, p. 91). The communication between those in the science field is highly reliant on rhetorical construction (Gross, 1990, p. 91). A historical look at the scientific view of the opioid crisis reveals the most current paradigmatic shifts as society grapples with the rhetorical constructs of addiction and addicts.

3.4 RHETORIC AND ADDICTION

There are two prevailing paradigms on addiction in America: addiction as a "moral failing" and addiction as "a brain-based disease" (U.S. Department of Health and Human Services & Centers for Disease Control and Prevention, 2016, p. v). With each paradigm comes drastically different opinions on how to handle the crisis. Those who believe addiction is a moral failing believe in the *criminal justice model* (U.S. Department of Health and Human Services & Centers for Disease Control and Prevention, 2016, p. 1–2). In this model, discipline and punish, such as longer jail times and stricter laws, are used to try to solve the issue. *The Surgeon General's Report on Alcohol, Drugs, and Health* concludes this model is not effective at stopping addiction and "continues to rob the United States of its most valued asset—people." The millions of people still suffering with addiction after numerous encounters with the justice system are evidence of the criminal justice model's failure (U.S. Department of Health and Human Services & Centers for Disease Control and Prevention, 2016, p. 1–2). Yet, on November 29, 2017, Attorney General Jeff Sessions announced he had allocated money for funding police officers to combat the opioid crisis, relying on the criminal justice model to prosecute opioid addicts (Cunningham, 2017, p. 1). "The emphasis continues to be punishment, so I think it's very concerning," said Gabrielle de la Gueronniere, director of policy for the Legal Action Center, a nonprofit organization that fights discrimination against people with a history of addiction. "We're not really treating this as an illness. There's a huge treatment gap," de la Gueronniere said (Cunningham, 2017, p. 1). It is notable that Murthy, under the Obama administration, put forth his recommendations relying on the "addiction as an illness" paradigm and that Jeff Sessions, under the Trump administration, is relying on the "criminal justice" model to prosecute addicts.

> The United States spends approximately $15 billion a year fighting illegal drugs, often on foreign soil. But America's deadliest drug epidemic begins and ends at home. More than 15,000 Americans now die annually after overdosing on prescription painkillers called opioids, according to the Centers for Disease Control and Prevention—more than from heroin, cocaine, and all other illegal drugs combined. (Catan et al., 2013, p. 123)

Also, because opioid prescriptions typically commence as a legal transaction, prosecution is difficult. The criminal justice model is expensive and has not proved to be effective.

Another of the many hindrances to the "discipline and punish" model is the stigma attached to admitting to being an addict. The etymology of the word "addict" is based in ancient Greek culture. Sociologist Erving Goffman explains the term "stigma" refers to bodily signs designed to expose something unusual and bad about the moral status of the "signifier" (Goffman, 1963, p. 1). In antiquity, signs indicating a person was "bad" or "unusual" were cut or burnt into the signifier's skin, usually in the case of "a slave, a criminal, or a traitor—a blemished person, ritually polluted, to be avoided especially in public places" (Goffman, 1963, p. 1). Later, in the Middle Ages, "two layers of metaphor were added to the term: the first referred to bodily signs of holy grace that took the form of eruptive blossoms on the skin; the second, a medical allusion to this religious allusion, referred to bodily signs" (Goffman, 1963, p. 1). In modern times, stigma involves social settings and attempting to establish categories in routine social interaction (Goffman, 1963, p. 1–3). Garb, appearance, occupation, and social status contribute to social identity to which normative expectations become a stigma (Goffman,

1963, p. 2). Stigmas are constructed from prejudices and inherent bias (Gadamer, 1989).

Opioids and stigma have a historical connection dating back to the late 1800s and early 1900s in China as "citizens who appeared normal and exhibited no criminal or socially stigmatized behavior before smoking opium were darkly transformed into liars, swindlers, thieves, robbers, muggers, pickpockets, beggars, prostitutes and ne'er-do-wells" (Slack, 2001, p. 43). Opium smokers historically became stigmatized as they shifted from the "casual" smoker for pleasure to a full-blown addict engaging in deviant behaviors. The negative and "immoral" stigma in the Chinese society extended to those who profited from the opium sales. Warlords, jianshang (wicked merchants), secret society members, and gangsters were seen as evil and disgraceful to society (Slack, 2001, p. 43–45). Profiting from the opium epidemic in the nineteenth and twentieth century in China was seen as evil and immoral.

Goffman notes that stigma today relates more to disgrace than to physical evidence and that stigmas create a way for society to establish a means of categorizing persons (Goffman, 1963, p. 2–3). Stigmas can create an impediment for treatment for addicts in the current historical moment. Murthy calls for an elimination of the stigmas associated with the brain-based disease of addiction, in the same way that common diseases, like diabetes and heart disease, lack stigma.

Some people may encounter an "enacted stigma" which occurs when a person directly experiences difficulty in, for example, obtaining employment, reduced options for housing, and interpersonal rejection due to stigma (Luoma et al., 2007, p. 1332). Olsen and Sharfstein (2014) explain conceptualizing opioid use disorder as a medical illness is often overshadowed by the misconception that opioid use disorder is a moral weakness or a willful choice.

People may also experience "self-stigma," or negative thoughts, such as shame and fear, that can arise from association with a stigmatized group (Luoma et al., 2007, p. 1332). The stigmas attached to the word "addict" present clinical challenges in having individuals openly seek treatment. The stigmas associated with the word "addict" have created "higher levels of secrecy coping" with the addiction and have been associated with many indicators of "poor functioning" (Luoma et al., 2007, p. 1331). Whether internalized or externalized, the stigma attached to addiction creates hurdles when seeking treatment. According to Stuart (2019) there are similar hurdles created between stigmas for substance use and mental health issues. Stuart (2019) explains mental health stigmas and substance use stigma create barriers to accessing evidence-based medication maintenance and other life-saving treatments.

The implications of "stigma" and the opioid crisis are that often negative stigmas are reinforced to popularize the "discipline and punish" paradigm. Stuart (2019) notes the physician community could be reinforcing these stereotypes when using pejorative language such as describing a positive drug screening as "dirty" or using the word "junkie" to describe a person with substance abuse disorder. In modernity, an addict may resort to deviance to tend to the addiction of opioids and thus be thought of as "a person who is quite thoroughly bad, or dangerous, or weak. He is thus reduced in our minds from a whole and usual person to a tainted, discounted one. Such an attribute is a stigma, especially when its discrediting effect is very extensive; sometimes it is also a failing, a handicap, or a short-coming" (Goffman," 1963, p. 3). This stigma is often relied upon in gaining public support for the discipline and punish model and, as Goffman predicts, is quite powerful.

Conversely, those in the scientific community who view addiction as a brain-based disease believe in exploring a "scientific evidence base for prevention, treatment, and recovery," thereby increasing investments in cognitive behavioral rehabilitation and pharmaceutical treatment (U.S. Department of Health and Human Services & Centers for Disease Control and Prevention, 2016, p. v). Murthy acknowledges the paradigmatic shift necessary to change public perceptions regarding addiction: "As the first-ever Surgeon General's Report on this important topic, [*The Surgeon General's Report on Alcohol, Drugs, and Health*] aims to shift the way our society thinks about substance misuse and substance use disorders while defining actions we can take to prevent and treat these conditions" (2016, p. V). Murthy continues to argue that this shift is necessary because addiction is no different from "heart disease, diabetes, and cancer" and should require the same level of medical attention (2016, p. V). Murthy's use of the term "shift" is reminiscent of Kuhn's paradigm shifts; Murthy is rhetorically constructing facts to make the shift occur. Murthy's report defines an addiction as "the most severe form of substance use disorder, associated with compulsive or uncontrolled use of one or more substances. Addiction is a chronic brain disease that has the potential for both recurrence (relapse) and recovery" (p. 1–6). The entire description of addiction is explained in a medical framework throughout the report, emphasizing that addiction is a disease that affects the brain.

Opioids, after all, cause long-lasting changes to the brain, "rewiring some areas to crave more drugs while simultaneously damaging the parts that can control those cravings" (Catan, 2013, p. 126). The drugs can "damage the brain's ability to feel pleasure, so regular users eventually need to take them not to get high or help with pain but just to feel normal"; thus, avoiding withdrawal symptoms often continues the cycle of opioid use (Catan, 2013, p. 126). The paradigm of "addiction as a brain-based disease" relies on medical jargon and, as an approach, seeks medical intervention to aid in curing the addiction. Notably, in the "addiction as a moral failing" paradigm, a person who enters the criminal justice system is known as a defendant while, in the "addiction as a brain based disease" model, the same person is referred to as a patient.

Addiction, or a substance use disorder, is "a medical illness caused by repeated misuse of a substance or substances" (U.S. Department of Health and Human Services & Centers for Disease Control and Prevention, 2016, p. 1–6). According to *The Surgeon General's Report*, citing the Diagnostic and Statistic Manual of Mental Disorders, fifth edition (DSM-5), "substance use disorders are characterized by clinically significant impairments in health, social function, and impaired control over substance use and are diagnosed through assessing cognitive, behavioral, and psychological symptoms. Substance use disorders range from mild to severe and from temporary to chronic" (p. 1–6). The paradigmatic shift from addiction as a moral failing to addiction as a disease brings a variety of new treatments for addiction. Taking medicine to control pharmaceutical addiction may seem counterintuitive, but pharmacological options exist: "Neurochemical systems involved in the transition from drug use to the compulsive use of addiction will provide the rational basis for development of pharmacotherapies for drug addiction" (Koob, 2000, p. 170). Methadone maintenance therapy (MMT), for instance, is considered a pharmacological option for opioid addiction (Ward et al., 1999, p. 221). MMT involves the daily administration of the oral opioid agonist methadone as a treatment for opioid dependence. Advocates for pharmacological treatment of addiction claim that "MMT improves health and reduces illicit heroin use, infectious-disease transmission, and overdose death" (Ward et al., 1999, p. 221). The paradigm for addiction treatment is currently amid a shift, from the scientific paradigm of "going cold-turkey" and experiencing painful withdrawal, to pharmacologically treating patients' addictions using methadone.

3.5 RHETORIC, PAIN, AND OPIOIDS

"Pain is among the most common complaints for which individuals seek medical attention," and, when individuals are in pain, they seek medical attention in the hopes their pain will be relieved (Savage et al., 2003, p. 655). Opioids are commonly used in moderate to severe pain management. Though opioid medications come in a myriad of forms and vary in their effectiveness, issues of tolerance, and dependence, addiction must be thoughtfully considered prior to treatment with any opioid (Inturrisi, 2002, p. S3). The use of opioids for pain relief is in crisis; the scientific community is questioning the paradigm of pharmacological prescription opioids.

The Interagency Guideline on Opioid Dosing for Chronic Non-cancer Pain (CNCP) (Agency Medical Directors Group, 2007) came out firmly against the overprescribing of opioids and issued a revision in 2010 with the following recommendations to physicians: First, try alternatives to opioids for pain, and then only the lowest dose should be prescribed; additionally, long-acting or controlled, release opioids (OxyContin, fentanyl patches, and methadone) should not be prescribed for acute pain (p. 1).

A randomized clinical trial including 240 people experiencing chronic back pain, chronic hip pain, or chronic knee osteoarthritis pain was published in the *Journal of the American Medical Association* in March 2018. The authors had affiliations with various medical school departments at the University of Minnesota and Indiana University, but also the Center for Health Information and Communication at Roudebush Veterans Affairs Medical Center in Indianapolis, Indiana (Krebs in Hilden, 2018, p. 872). Collaboration between medical doctors and scholars of health communication went into the study's planning and delivery of the results. This study was constructed "scientifically" and relied upon health communication strategies to "diffuse" the information.

The study divided the group into an opioid group and a nonopioid group. The opioid group received morphine, oxycodone, or hydrocodone/acetaminophen, and the nonopioid group received acetaminophen or a nonsteroidal anti-inflammatory drug (Krebs in Hilden, 2018, p. 872). The study, entitled the "Effect of Opioid vs Nonopioid Medications on Pain-Related Function in Patients with Chronic Back Pain or Hip or Knee Osteoarthritis Pain," found that "treatment with opioids was not superior to treatment with nonopioid medications for improving pain-related function over 12 months. Results do not support initiation of opioid therapy for moderate to severe chronic back pain or hip or knee osteoarthritis pain" (Krebs in Hilden, 2018, p. 872).

Furthermore, "no strong evidence-based" connection between opioids and relief of chronic non-cancer pain has been established (Kissin, 2013, p. 513). David Morris explores the construct of "pain" and why opioids may not be the best treatment for pain. Morris explains that, contrary to scientific belief in the recent past, there is more to pain than just "a particularly complex signal broadcast over nerves leading from the site of injury to the brain" (Morris, 1991, p. 1). Rather, pain is a multidimensional construct, and pain has historical roots, cultural applications for pain management, and psychosocial elements (Morris, 1991, p. 1–8). The United States has a culturally and historically constructed connection between "pain, doctors, ointments, pills, surgery, hospitals, labs, and insurance forms" (Morris, 1991, p. 2). Culture is what pulls people "irresistibly toward the medicine cabinet, as if pills and tablets held a kind of magnetic, eternal attraction for the unseen torments of a bad back or any other type of pain" (Morris, 1991, p. 2). In the current opioid crisis, marketing practices have created and constructed the connection between opioids and the relief of chronic pain; "this was all done with the cooperation and encouragement of pharmaceutical companies" (Hilden, 2018, p. 1). The link between large and powerful institutions like Purdue Pharma controlling the dominant episteme cannot be overlooked.

Morris (1991) asserts the remedy for pain is not always found in a bottle. Instead, pain can be best understood via listening to the voices on the margins of pain—patients, historical interpretations of those who managed pain in the past, doctors who practice alternative treatments—and reading about those who have managed their pain without opioids. Morris (1991) cites one particular example from Kant:

> Immanuel Kant, sitting up late at night in Konigsberg, at the end of the eighteenth century, with his toes glowing red from an excruciating attack of gout. Kant's method for dealing with his affliction was to concentrate with all his might on one object, no matter what. He would think, for example, of the Roman orator Cicero and of everything that could be thought in connection with the name of Cicero. Through this method he was so successful in banishing his pain that in the morning he sometimes wondered whether he had simply imagined it. True, Kant as a philosopher no doubt possessed unusual powers of concentration. The crucial point, however, is that he did not merely distract himself, as if watching a sitcom. Nor did he sit fretting about his health. He employed the full force of his mind. (p. 7)

Kant did not live in a historical moment where opioids were being overprescribed for pain; Morris's point is there are cultural assumptions about pain and how to manage it.

Americans live with the "Myth of Two Pains"—the myth that mental and physical pain are separate categories (Morris, 1991, p. 9). Morris concludes that mental pain can manifest physically and vice versa. He writes, "The pain of a stubbed toe obviously has a different immediate source than the pain of a no-holds-barred divorce. Yet, in the long run, different sources do not necessarily imply different pains" (Morris, 1991, p. 9). The Myth of Two Pains perpetuates the idea of pharmacologically treating pains for the body while treating the mind with different pharmacological options. Morris acknowledges that it is difficult "to demythologize our widespread cultural assumption that body and mind produce two utterly different kinds of pain" (Morris, 1991, p. 10). The idea that mental pain manifests physically has long been established as "a growing body of evidence suggests that biological mechanisms underlie a bidirectional link between mood disorders and many medical illnesses" (Evans et al., 2005, p. 175). Studies have supported the mind-body connection, such as the finding that "comorbid depressive-anxiety disorder

[is] more strongly associated with several physical conditions" (Scott et al., 2007, p. 117). Heart disease and chronic pain conditions show the strongest associations with depressive and anxiety disorders, which is consistent with research highlighting the robust links between these physical conditions and major depressive disorder (Evans et al., 2005, p. 188). Therefore, pain is not simply a "medical" problem involving nerves; pain engages personal traumas, complex cultural constructs, and biological processes of living.

A society's experience of pain and how pain is managed is influenced by the historical moment and culture (Morris, 1991, p. 1–15). "Our culture—the modern, Western, industrial, technocratic world—has succeeded in persuading us that pain is simply and entirely a medical problem" (Morris, 1991, p. 1). Pain is a construct or, according to Morris, an "experience" that brings about certain behaviors and attitudes that can produce more pain. Pain can create a negative feedback loop whereby pain brings about social isolation, and in turn social isolation creates more pain. When a person becomes isolated from supportive loved ones and communication, the person's physical health problems can intensify (Eisenberger, 2012, p. 421). The "Myth of Two Pains," or the inability to separate emotional pain from physical pain, is relevant when considering a remedy for pain (Morris, 1991, p. 9–12). Morris (1991) explains, "Less obviously, pain, too, places us within a social world where what we feel cannot be easily disentangled from what we learn from our culture and from how other people respond to us. Pain may keep us from working, push us into the role of invalid, drive away friends, and wall us up in a personal prison of isolation" (p. 14). The way a culture manages pain becomes the invisible teacher for how one copes with pain (Morris, 1991). Being perceived as sick and in pain in Western culture often leads to further isolation as "healthy people" are often made uncomfortable by the sick and by those in pain (Jackson, 2000, p. 145–147).

In this historical moment in the West, there is emphasis placed on the mind/body distinction (Jackson, 2000, p. 145). Jackson explains the way patients describe their pain to a doctor impacts how the pain is managed. Jackson writes, "Someone who believes her pain is due to a physical cause (e.g., angina produced by hardened arteries) will probably experience a pain in the region of the heart differently from a pain she believes to be emotional in origin (e.g., heartache caused by unrequited love)" (Jackson, 2000, p. 145).

Stigma and emotional pain are also explored. People in Western culture may not admit to emotional pain in the hopes of not "seeming weak" (Galanti, 2014, p. 66). Stigma is of particular concern to many pain sufferers. The stigma that accompanies pain that is seen to be emotionally caused and does not go away, such as emotional heartache, "draws disapproval if it does not diminish in time: the sufferer should 'get over it' after a while. A clinician's diagnosis of such a pain would probably seem stigmatizing to the sufferer"

(Jackson, 2000, p. 145). Hence, etymology of the source of the pain and experience of the sensations of pain are related. The sufferer's belief about the cause of the pain will almost always have an effect on the experience, cause, and the embodiment of the sensation of pain, and response to the treatment of pain (Jackson, 2000, p. 145).

An example of how pain is being managed in the current historical moment is highlighted in the story of a woman named Jaclyn Kinkade. At 23 years old, Kinkade was found dead in her home in Florida, killed by the pills she was taking to alleviate her back pain and neck pain (Catan, 2013, p. 123). The doctor she worked for as a receptionist first prescribed Kinkade the opioid Endocet, a drug containing oxycodone, in October 2006 (Catan, 2013, p. 127). In a diary entry, Kinkade writes, "I'd never taken opioids before, but I started the med routine and OMG I felt no pain." (Catan, 2013, p. 127). Kinkade quickly became addicted to the opioids and began to visit pain clinics in her area, seeking multiple doctors willing to write prescriptions for her pain. In a few short years, she lost her job, her boyfriend, and her parents' trust; the addiction to opioids robbed her of her life (Catan, 2013, p. 123–131). Kinkade's quest to "feel no pain" led to her own death.

But is feeling no pain a worthwhile goal? Morris, seeking to understand life without pain, finds an answer far from what might be expected. Morris (1991) writes about Edward Gibson, who was born with a rare disorder making him unable to feel the sensation of pain (p. 14). The inability to feel pain turned out to be more of a curse than a blessing. Gibson performed shows sticking needles through his cheeks and allowing audience members to stick needles into his skin. Gibson's inability to feel pain made him a "spectacle" and kept him from relating to people around him. Morris (1991) states, "A pain-free life for Edward Gibson proved to be a meaningless benefit that left him more or less indifferent" (p. 13). Pain is a part of life; not being able to experience pain is a dangerous existence. Morris writes that children who do not experience pain and are very likely to get hurt and even live shorter lives (Morris, 1991, p. 12–14). Imagine jumping from the top of a slide to the ground, or directly off a cliff as a child, and feeling no pain. Such experiences, however, are likely to bring grave injury. Pain teaches people how to survive and avoid injuries. The anticipatory sensation of pain prevents people from engaging in high-risk behaviors. Pain serves a purpose and creates meaning. According to Morris (1991), "the words pain and meaning serve an indispensable social function precisely because they cannot be easily pinned down" (p. 17). How people interpret and begin to make sense of crises and loss of life begins with a constructive hermeneutic approach, allowing multiple understandings of this historical moment's response to pain.

3.6 FRAMING

According to Rettie (2004), "Frames are not mental objects, but concepts used to decipher what is happening around us" (p. 117). The current historical moment provides one such frame for interpretation. Looking to theory may help in understanding how the opioid crisis has been framed. Gadamer (1989) explains in *Truth and Method* that meaning and interpretation are not fixed points on a horizon; rather, there is room for multiple interpretations, and several points on a horizon of meaning have validity. In other words, there is room for multiple interpretations because the way one understands and interprets is based on bias, prejudices, previous life experiences, and historical moments that shape the lens through which one sees the world. In this section, I use Gadamer's concept of horizon of meanings to explain a constructive hermeneutical approach.

First, a constructive hermeneutical approach understands that people have intrinsic biases and prejudices from which they cannot separate (Gadamer, 1989, p. 280). Second, as a situation or text is analyzed, elements of *strangeness* and *familiarity* emerge (Gadamer, 1989, p. 259). Gadamer explains constructive hermeneutics through the metaphors of *strangeness and familiarity* and the polarity that shifts between the two concepts (Gadamer, 1989, p. 259). The locus of understanding a text is the shifting that occurs between these two poles; a situation that once appeared strange begins to make sense and become familiar. One way to begin to make sense of something strange is to try to answer the question "what is going on here?" When interpreting the situation, it may be helpful to view actions as part of a schemata and through frames (Goffman, 1974, p. 1–15).

Interpreting a crisis must begin at some arbitrary point. Goffman's theory of framing analysis is one way to begin to frame the opioid crisis. A frame focuses on a particular element of a particular scenario to prevent getting lost in a menagerie of ideas. In *Frame Analysis*, Goffman (1974) develops his theory using the insights of William James, Alfred Schutz, and Gregory Bateson. Frame analysis begins by considering the very broad question "what is it that's going on here?" although that question can create a bias toward a unitary moment in time and may guide perspective to a unitary event (Goffman, 1974, p. 9). However, bias is necessary for interpreting life. Goffman claims, "My aim is to try to isolate some of the basic frameworks of understanding available in our society for making sense out of events and to analyze the special vulnerabilities to which these frames of reference are subject" (Goffman, 1974, p. 10). According to Goffman, understanding "what is going on here" requires a firm grasp of the ideas of perspective and point of view.

Frame analysis allows for an organization of experience, but the analysis needs a starting point. One such starting point can be a "strip," which is a "raw batch of occurrences" (Goffman, 1974, p. 10). Then, the frame analysis provides assumptions about what is going on. Goffman (1974) writes "observers actively project their frames of reference on the world immediately around them" (p. 39). Frames provide the contexts that enable interpretation of events. The same section or "strip" of experience can take different frames. For instance, an event understood at first as a marriage ceremony may be reframed as a rehearsal (Rettie, 2004, p. 117). Culture and the historical moment ground interpretation as "frames are socially shared and culture-specific" (Rettie, 2004, p. 117). Fairhurst and Sarr write about the importance of framing in both the creation of meaning and in the interpretative process of understanding: "Frames exert their power not only through what they highlight but also through what they leave out" (Fairhurst and Sarr, 1996, p. 4). When "creat[ing] a bias towards one interpretation," some aspects are highlighted while others are excluded (Fairhurst and Sarr, 1996, p. 4).

3.7 CONCLUSIONS AND CONNECTIONS BETWEEN THE FRAME AND THE OPIOID CRISIS

The essential tool in the creation of meaning is the ability to frame (Fairhurst and Sarr, 1996, p. 1–10). Fairhust and Sarr note that the frame helps to decipher the meaning of a subject, to make sense of it, to judge its character and significance (p. 3). To see the addict as a defendant through the criminal justice model, or to view the addict as a patient in the model of addiction as a brain-based illness, is based on framing. Focusing on the changing brain chemistry and medical jargon implies a choice of "one particular meaning or set of meanings over another" (Fairhurst and Sarr, 1996, p. 3). The frame allows one to interpret and allows a person to focus on shifting the strange and making sense of it, transforming it to the familiar. Hence, seeing addiction as medical condition.

The patient's point of view is its own frame, as well. When a patient is suffering from emotional pain that manifests physically, the patient may choose a frame that focuses only on the physical pain. This frame neglects the underlying emotions as the patient seeks to relieve the pain with pills. Similarly, framing can be used from a doctor's point of view. A doctor may have financial incentives or an ongoing treatment plan that frames the patient's course of treatment. There are several pain societies that have framed opioid prescribing and opioid usage in ways that very much favor the pharmaceutical industries (Lembke, 2016, p. 63).

Fairhurst and Sarr explain how framing is fundamental to goal achievement (1996, p. 24). Framing is relevant in "setting our communication goals, whether they revolve around tasks, relationships, or identities, we are making choices" (Fairhurst and Sarr, 1996, p. 24). Framing techniques and reaching goals originates from the work of Robert Mager, who introduced the theory of "goal analysis." The logic behind goal analysis is to narrow the set of possible meanings for a broad goal and thus pave a more direct path to achieving the goal (Mager, 1972, p. 1–8). Mager distinguishes between "fuzzies" and performances. Fuzzies are abstract and not easily understood; for example, "I want to do a good job" is a fuzzie. Performance is based in specific terms to meet a goal; for example, "I want to sell 100 widgets" (Mager, 1972). The concepts of intentionality and specific action in the framing process that Big Pharma (the global pharmaceutical industry) employed to convince physicians to overprescribe were based on specific performances or planned presentations at medical conferences across the country (Lembke, 2016, p. 60–70). The purpose of this chapter is to argue a new paradigm in opioid management has been constructed. Paradigm shifts result in scientific revolutions. In the past decade, a new paradigm has been constructed that stresses opioid therapy is not appropriate for chronic pain and conservative opioid therapy is safer than liberal prescribing. In the 1990s, efforts to improve treatment of pain using opioids failed to take into account opioids' addictiveness and lack of documented effectiveness in the treatment of chronic pain, and the old paradigm of liberal opioid prescribing was questioned by many in the scientific community (Frieden and Houry, 2016). The next chapter examines in detail the framing techniques employed by various professions and professional organizations.

In the next chapter, I will explore Goffman's question of "what is going on here?" regarding the professionals who have contributed to the severity of the opioid crisis. More specifically, understanding the role of the professions and what can occur when professional ethics are violated.

Chapter Four

Protecting the Professions—Doctor Versus Drug Dealer

4.1 INTRODUCTION

This chapter looks to the literature on what occurs when a profession becomes threatened by crisis. *Professional Civility,* by Fritz (2013), outlines what it means to be a "professional" and what role the professional plays in protecting the *home* for the professions. This chapter highlights stories of professionals who have not been stewards of professional ideals and how their actions have affected the medical profession. Also, I explore the history of pain as the fifth vital, and the concept of "pain medicine." What is a pain doctor? How is this profession framed as appropriate or inappropriate in the literature? Additionally, this chapter considers the multifaceted question of how the opioid crisis began in the United States. I look to branding techniques used by drug manufacturers or drug detailers, accreditation organizations, and physician specialty societies, as appropriate, and include the concept of "patient-directed" care such as Press-Ganey and other organizations that survey patient satisfaction.

4.2 VIOLATIONS OF PROFESSIONAL JUDGMENT

Health professionals and health organizations (i.e., drug manufacturer and physician societies) are two groups that have contributed to the opioid crisis. It appears that doctors abusing opioid prescribing is not the exception but more of the norm; an investigation conducted by National Public Radio (NPR) found that doctors, dentists, and other health care providers still prescribe highly addictive pain medications at rates widely considered unsafe (Mann, 2020). Patients in 2020 received more than twice the volume of opioids considered normal before the prescribing boom began in the late 1990s (Mann, 2020). Professional judgement is called into question when, "We're [United States] 5% of the world's population, but we consume 80% of the world's prescription opioids," said Dr. Jonathan Chen, a physician and researcher at Stanford University Medical Center who studies prescribing patterns (Chen in Mann, 2020). The professional ideal may be being violated more than most people realize and doctors are engaging in unprofessional and illegal behaviors.

There are extreme and illegal examples of betrayal of the professional ideal. Five prominent doctors in New York were recently arrested for taking bribes of at least $100,000 each to prescribe Subsys (Weiser and Thomas, 2018). The doctors were bribed through an extravagant "speaker program" of "fake educational events, often at luxurious venues and sometimes involving only the paid physician speaker and an Insys sales representative" (Dyer, 2016, p. 355). Subsys is a spray form of the highly addictive fentanyl and is made by Insys Therapeutics (Dyer, 2016, p. 355; Weiser and Thomas, 2018). "These prominent doctors swore a solemn oath to place their patients' care above all else," said Geoffrey S. Berman, the U.S. attorney for the Southern District of New York. "Instead, they engaged in a malignant scheme to prescribe fentanyl, a dangerous and potentially fatal narcotic 50 to 100 times more potent than morphine, in exchange for bribes in the form of speaker fees" (Berman in Weiser and Thomas, 2018). The opioid crisis began with a violation of the "professional ideal" and the lack of attention on addiction, ethics, and morals by several in the medical profession (Lembke, 2016). Thus, this section seeks to understand the connection between the opioid crisis and doctors, pharmaceutical company executives, and pain societies who betrayed the "professional ideal."

Dr. Anna Lembke (2016) highlights problems in the medical profession and their connections to the opioid crisis in her book *Drug Dealer, MD: How Doctors Were Duped, Patients Got Hooked, and Why It's So Hard to Stop.* Dr. Lembke received her medical degree from Stanford University, is on the faculty of the Stanford University School of Medicine, and is a diplomat of both the American Board of Psychiatry and Neurology and the American Board of Addiction Medicine (*Anna Lembke*, 2017). She has published over 50 peer-reviewed articles, chapters, and commentaries, including in *The New England Journal of Medicine*, *The Journal of the American Medical Association*, the *Journal of General Internal Medicine*, and *Addiction* (*Anna Lembke*, 2017).

Dr. Lembke provides an insider perspective into the medical profession and the ethical violations and abuses of power taking place in hospitals and doctors' offices across the nation, putting the professional ideal into question.

Lembke (2016) writes in the prologue of *Drug Dealer, MD* about a woman under her care in the hospital while suffering from nonspecific low back pain (p. 1–10). The patient, screaming out in pain, treating the nurses poorly, demands more opioids to treat the pain. The patient's life is plagued with dysfunction and poor relationships (Lembke, 2016, p. 1–10). Dr. Lembke (2016) diagnosed the patient with opioid addiction and suggests an opioid tapering schedule to slowly detox as the patient has been prescribed "1,200 different opioid pills obtained from sixteen different doctors" in the months prior to her admission (p. 3). Lembke also recommended an addiction recovery center once the patient was released from the hospital.

But Lembke's colleagues ignored her orders to stop giving the patient opioids because the patient threatened legal action against them for leaving her in pain; moreover, Lembke's colleagues continued to prescribe high-dose opioids for the remainder of her hospitalization and subsequent hospitalizations (Lembke, 2016). When doctors continue to prescribe high doses of opioids despite a clear addiction issue, they call into question their own professional judgment or lack thereof (Lembke, 2016, p. 115–131).

Dr. Lembke's experience is representative of what is occurring across the United States. "It's possible some clinicians just simply aren't aware of existing evidence-based recommendations," said Christina Mikosz, one of the CDC's lead researchers studying opioid prescribing. "The other possibility is that they are aware, and they just choose not to follow them" (Mikosz in Mann, 2020). Lembke (2016) explains the patient who was receiving high-dose opioids mentioned in the prologue of her book was emblematic of a new normal. On November 1, 2011, the Centers for Disease Control and Prevention (CDC), declared a "prescription drug epidemic"; and the CDC was unequivocal about what had caused this epidemic: "prescription opioid painkillers and psychotherapeutic drugs being prescribed more widely by physicians" (Lembke, 2016, p. 4). Thus, creating a precarious situation in the United States, approximately 4,000 deaths involving opioid painkillers were reported in 1999, and this multiplied by a factor of four to 16,235 deaths in 2013 (Lembke, 2016). Opioid painkillers like OxyContin mixed with sedative benzodiazepines contributed to many of the overdose deaths (Lembke, 2016). Lembke (2016) is clear that medical doctors are at fault in this crisis as they overprescribe opioids: "Prescribers wrote enough opioid prescriptions in 2012 to medicate every American adult around the clock for a month" (p. 4). Doctors' professional judgment is called into question when exploring these issues. Should doctors write prescriptions just because they can? Or should doctors adhere to the professional ideal and refuse to write prescriptions if the prescription might do more harm than good?

4.3 WHAT IS A PROFESSIONAL? WHAT IS A PROFESSION?

In "The True Professional Ideal in America," Kimball (1996) examines the word *profession* from a historical context and seeks to understand the *episodic changes* associated with the word (p. 2–6). The *episodic changes* are changes during historical time periods. "Theology, law, medicine, and education originally became associated in the medieval universities, which provided people the meeting ground for learning," and these four professions have been referred to as "the four great traditional professions" (Kimball, 1996, p. 6). Into the fifteenth century, theology was the highest esteemed profession. In the sixteenth and seventeenth centuries, early American colonies such as New Jersey granted exemptions for military duty to ministers, doctors, school masters, and civil officers, carving out a level of respect for those professions (Kimball, 1996, p. 6). In the nineteenth and twentieth centuries, professions in the science field gained respect and a prominent place in society. For example, "in 1876, the noted astronomer Simon Newcomb call[s] upon Americans to establish their greatness by pursuing science"; in 1898, W. J. McGee states, "America has become a nation of science" (Kimball, 1996, p. 203). Kimball writes that people who study science are respected: "The man of science appeared in the second half of the nineteenth century as 'a special breed' having cultural authority (Kimball, 1996, p. 203). A "religion of science" became popular with intellectuals as science gained prominence (Kimball, 1996, p. 203). Professionals in the scientific fields, specifically medicine, are valued in society; they help people who are in pain, with the goal of restoring health.

In the current historical moment, the "professions represent a wide variety of occupations engaged in specialized knowledge work in the service economy," and typically involve support staff and other professionals who aid in the completion of a work product (Fritz, 2013, p. 4). According to Sullivan, the word "profession" and the ideal of a professional bestows an associated level of prestige "as professions are high-status occupations that bring power and privilege to their members" (Fritz, 2013, p. 5). There have been shifts with archetypes of the professions, which now include an "extended set of occupations," yet all professionals have a reasonable amount of autonomy, based on a specialized knowledge base, and an adherence to ethical norms in both their professional and personal lives (Fritz, 2013, p. 5). "Ethical norms provide a basis for self-evaluation of professions as communities of practice, defining the 'good' that is protected and promoted by a given profession" (Fritz, 2013, p. 5). A good, as defined by Arnett, Fritz, and Bell (2008), "is a central value or set of values manifested in communicative practices that we seek to protect and promote in our discourse together" (p. 2). The *professional ideal* is the good professions seek to uphold. The *professional ideal* includes ethical practices with others in the profession, professionals in different fields, community members, and perhaps themselves (Fritz, 2013). The telos of a profession is productivity, and "productivity permits the organization to thrive and contributes to the realization of the good of persons as contributing beings" (Fritz, 2013, p. 58). The professions and practicing professionals "contribute to the good of human flourishing" when there is an embodiment of the "professional ideal" through the engagement of professional practice with the other (Fritz, 2013, p. 46). The *professional ideal* requires adhering to an ethical framework; however, greed cannot be overlooked when considering professions.

In addition to Fritz's assertion that greed must be considered when exploring the professions, Giddens expands upon this notion in regard to the sciences, technology, and expertise. Giddens explores the notion of modernity and the lack of emphasis placed upon morality and ethics when considering a scientific outlook (Giddens, 2013, p. 8). The professional, engaging in the performance of the profession, has been entrusted to act in the best interest of their clients, patients, and students, among others (Fritz, 2013, p. 46). The opioid crisis brings to the surface what occurs when the professional violates the "professional ideal."

Therefore, it is important to ask what happens when a profession is called into question for a severe violation of ethics. The next section addresses the historical moment whereby the profession of medicine is called into question for doctors violating professional standards. I then seek to understand how this violation of ethical standards has contributed to the opioid crisis.

4.4 THE ETHIC OF MEDICINE AND DOCTORS WHO BETRAY THE ETHIC

The topic of medical ethics is multidimensional and dynamic. Dubois (2005) writes, "Ethics in the medical world and, more specifically, in pain medicine, is, by and large, a roadmap that allows us (doctors) to keep practicing in the face of an increasingly complex—and often confusing and contradictory—environment without losing our way and ending in bedlam, jail, or forced retirement" (p. 201). There is no doubt that medical ethics is controversial, but "some sort of guidelines or laws for practicing morally acceptable medicine have existed for at least 4,000 years" (Dubois, 2005, p. 201). The Hippocratic Oath, especially, has existed up to "modern times as a principle of moral behavior in medicine" (Dubois, 2005, p. 201).

The Oath or, as it is commonly called, the Hippocratic Oath was written in about 400 (BCE) and is one of the oldest binding documents in history (Miles, 2005; Tyson, 2001). The Oath provides an ethical framework for doctors by listing specific principles or ideals for the medical profession to adhere to when treating patients both rich and poor, free man and slave alike (Miles, 2005, p. 2; Tyson, 2001, p. 3). The author of the Oath is not known with any degree of certainty, nor is the exact context for which it was written, known although it is believed to have been used in Antiquity to swear in medical apprentices (Miles, 2005, p. 3). Miles (2005) argues, "The Oath addresses perennial issues for medical ethics. I believe that it speaks to us still" (p. 5). The Oath is important when considering the professional ethic and the professional ideal. Medical students take the Oath, or a version of the Oath, upon graduation from medical school (Tyson, 2001).

One ethical ideal from the Oath is "And I will use regimens for the benefit of the ill in accordance with my ability and my judgment, but from what is it to their harm or injustice I will keep them" (Miles, 2005, p. XIII). Doctors are entrusted with maintaining health or restoring health, and that begs the question whether doctors are, through lack of judgment, overprescribing and inflicting harm. Lembke (2016) writes, "By 2010, for the first time in history, unintentional drug poisonings represented the leading cause of injury death in the United States, exceeding deaths due to car accidents. The total toll of prescription opioid overdoses between 1999 and 2013 exceeded 175,000 lives" (p. 4). Patients are visiting doctors to relieve pain, and doctors are prescribing opioids to relieve pain at alarming rates. Harm is being done to the profession of medicine as harm is being inflicted on patients. Kovacs, Gilbert, and Oetgen (2020) explore the delicate balance between wanting to relieve patients' pain while simultaneously attempting to not create or worsen an opioid addiction.

Not only are there ethical implications, but this clear disregard for professional judgment also has criminal implications. Dr. Alan Arnold Godofsky, 61, of Ohio, "was found guilty of five counts of distributing oxycodone outside the scope of professional medical practice and not for a legitimate medical purpose" (Brookbank, 2017, p. 1). Dr. Godofsky has failed the professional ideal and has failed to adhere to a professional ethic. Shier says, "Sadly, this case represents yet another example of a physician abdicating his professional responsibility to his patients, placing his own profit over sound medical judgment, and fueling the opioid epidemic" (Brookbank, 2017). Lembke (2016) summarizes this failure to uphold professional ethics: "Doctors more interested in money than in the well-being of their patients took advantage of the rising demand for opioid painkillers in the 1990s and 2000s as a way to get rich quick" (p. 117). Doctors whose actions are perpetuating the crisis are behaving unethically and illegally.

This crisis spread throughout the United States. Dr. Patel of Elko, Nevada, for example, deceived patients by showing them *fraudulent X-rays*, misleading patients to believe they had coronary issues that needed to be treated by him (U.S. Attorney's Office, 2017). Patel also "is accused of routinely prescribing fentanyl, hydrocodone, and oxycodone for his patients without a legitimate medical purpose from May 2014 to September 2017" (U.S. Attorney's Office, 2017). FBI Agent Aaron Rouse says, "Despite his physician's oath to do no harm, Dr. Patel recklessly prescribed opioids, for no legitimate medical purpose" (U.S. Attorney's Office, 2017). Patel's patients would quickly become addicted and return for numerous visits to get more prescriptions.

Though written in antiquity, the Hippocratic Oath foresees timeless issues such as romantic relationships influencing doctors' behaviors. The Hippocratic Oath states, "Into as many houses as I may enter, I will go for the benefit of the ill, while being far from all voluntary and destructive injustice, especially from sexual acts both upon women's bodies and upon men's, both of the free and of the slaves" (Miles, 2005, p. XIV). The ethical issues of personal relationships and treating relationships, especially when treating with opioids, are clear: The two shall not mix. Pennsylvania Attorney General Josh Shapiro announced criminal charges against Dr. Kenneth Cherry, an orthopedic surgeon in State College, Pennsylvania, "who wrote 63 prescriptions for opioid pain medications and other drugs to a woman who was not his patient, but with whom he was having an affair" (Kolesar, 2017, p. 1). The woman with whom he had an affair indicated having a "personal/sexual relationship" with Dr. Cherry, "and the doctor would write her prescriptions for pain medications and leave them in his unlocked car or truck for her to pick up" (Kolesar, 2017, p. 1). The medical profession is granted the autonomy to prescribe responsibly and without prejudice or bias; the romantic nature of this relationship created a strong bias, violating ethical lines.

These accounts about the prevalence of overprescribing and clearly illegal prescribing may force one to ask, "How did society get to this point?" Different physicians provide different explanations for the lack of ethical adherence in the medical profession. The dynamic nature of medicine—what is right today may be wrong tomorrow—complicates medical ethics, but medical ethics is worthy of study (Dubois, 2005, p. 202). Dr. Miles (2005) explains the majority of U.S. medical schools incorporate an oath into ceremonies for medical students, but "only one [school] uses a complete translation of the Oath," and others use an abridged version of the Oath or some other oath (p. 4). Most notably, only a dozen medical schools expose students to the Oath during medical ethics training (Miles, 2005, p. 4). Dr. Dubois adds that the myriad medical technologies invented in the second half of the twentieth century create "puzzling clinical situations" and that "old references to traditional moral authority [have] crumbled" (p. 201). The relatively new specialty of pain medicine developed an "Ethics Forum" in 2000 to attempt to look at the ethics of pain management (Dubois, 2005, p. 202). The next section seeks to understand the definition and role of pain doctors and the ethical issues attached to the specialty.

4.5 PAIN DOCTORS, PAIN SOCIETIES, AND THE FRAMING OF OPIOIDS

Pain is a biological, social, and cultural construct (Morris, 1998, p. 1–10). Furthermore, the choice to cope with pain, attempt to eliminate it with opioids, find meaning in the pain, or turn to an alternative to opioids such as acetaminophen, ibuprofen, acupuncture, or massage therapy, is also relevant to biological, cultural, and social factors (Morris, 1998, p. 1–16). How one chooses to *frame* pain and the management of pain can also be determined by bias or agendas (Lembke, 2016, p. 56–72). Recall from the last chapter how Fairhurst and Sarr (1996) describe the importance of framing in both the creation of meaning and the interpretative process of understanding: "Frames exert their power not only through what they highlight but also through what they leave out" (p. 4). When "creat[ing] a bias towards one interpretation," some aspects of an issue are highlighted while others are excluded (Fairhurst and Sarr, 1996, p. 4). This section focuses on pain societies' and the pharmaceutical industry's "framing" of opioid prescribing as a remedy for chronic pain.

Pain societies have defined pain in an attempt to have consistency of terminology in academic literature. The International Association for the Study of Pain, founded in 1973, "appoint[ed] a Subcommittee on Taxonomy charged with creating a definition [of pain] suitable for scientific discourse. This subcommittee consisted of fourteen of the most distinguished pain specialists in the world" (Morris, 1998, p. 16). The subcommittee of pain experts concluded pain is "an unpleasant sensory and emotional experience associated with actual or potential tissue damage or described in terms of such damage" (Morris, 1998, p. 16). Morris (1998) notes pain is an experience and not merely a sensation.

The specialty of pain medicine consists of a group of physicians whose sole focus is to manage pain. According to the American Society of Regional Anesthesia and Pain Medicine (n.d.), "A pain management specialist is a physician with special training in evaluation, diagnosis, and treatment of all different types of pain." There are three categories of pain: acute, chronic, and cancer. "Acute pain," the Mayo Clinic explains, "is a severe or sudden pain that resolves within a certain amount of time. You might feel acute pain when you have an illness, injury or surgery" (*Understanding Pain*, 2016). Chronic pain "is persistent, lasting for months or even longer. Chronic pain is considered a health condition in itself" (*Understanding Pain*, 2016). Cancer pain is most often caused by the cancer itself, often by a tumor pressing on bones, nerves, or organs (The American Cancer Society Medical and Editorial Content Team, 2019). It is important to note that the focus of this work is the rhetorical framing of opioids as a remedy for chronic pain.

Medical societies exist to support medical professions to promote the specialty and represent its doctors and also, in theory, to advocate for patients (Lembke, 2016). Opioids were once prescribed *sparingly* and mostly for acute pain, but, in the 1980s, pain societies began to advocate on behalf of pain doctors and pain patients for a more *liberal use of opioid painkillers* to treat chronic pain (Lembke, 2016). The pain societies campaigned to cure "*opiophobia*" by removing the stigma associated with taking and prescribing opioids and attaching a stigma to doctors who refuse to prescribe opioids (Lembke, 2016, p. 62).

The American Pain Society was founded in 1995, and their "self-proclaimed goal was to cure the medical community of 'opiophobia' [fear of prescribing opioids]" (Lembke, 2016, p. 63). I assert an "episodic shift" (Kimball, 1996, p. 2–5) occurred in the medical profession in 1995, when the American Pain Society was formed with the goal of curing "opiophobia," as physicians were persuaded that liberally prescribing opioids was best for their patients and thus changed their prescribing behavior. Additionally, I assert an "episodic shift" occurred in the medical profession when several pharmaceutical companies employed aggressive marketing techniques to frame opioids as the appropriate remedy for chronic pain (U.S. General Accounting Office [GAO], 2003, p. 4–28). Kimball explains rhetoric must be taken seriously when considering cultural transformations in the medical profession (Kimball, 1996, p. 6). Medical societies' rhetoric has influenced the behavior of their members (Lembke, 2016, p. 55–65). Specifically, Purdue Pharma's (manufacturer of OxyContin) rhetoric has influenced proprescribing behaviors in doctors and protreatment for patients (GAO, 2003, p. 4–28).

The American Pain Society and other pain societies succeeded in spreading pro-opioid prescribing rhetoric, the actions and financial involvement of the pharmaceutical industry or Big Pharma, academic physicians, and regulatory agencies all aided in this success (Lembke, 2016, p. 57). The medical societies with Big Pharma's financial backing have created campaigns to influence behavior, using doctors referred to as *thought leaders* to influence the average physician (Lembke, 2016, p. 58). *Thought leaders*, as they are called by Purdue Pharma, are doctors paid by the pharmaceutical industry (Lembke, 2016, p. 58). These thought leaders have traveled the country, speaking at medical conferences in support of certain drugs, especially opioids (Lembke, 2016, p. 58). The U.S. General Accounting Office (2003) has also noted the use of medical conferences to spread acceptance for opioids: "During the first 5 years that OxyContin was marketed, Purdue conducted over 40 national pain management and speaker training conferences, usually in resort locations such as Boca Raton, Florida, and Scottsdale, Arizona, to recruit and train health care practitioners for its national speaker bureau" (22). These trained speakers gave lectures about the "appropriate use of opioids, including oxycodone, the active ingredient in OxyContin, to their colleagues in various settings, such as local medical conferences and grand round presentations in hospitals involving physicians, residents, and interns" (GAO, 2003, p. 22). The subtly of Big Pharma's involvement is best explained as insidious:

> Pharmaceutical companies were careful not to overtly associate their thought leader's message with their brand. They often paid thought leaders large sums of money to speak, and in some instances provided the funds to subsidize the entire medical conference/seminar. They promoted the drug company's product, while also furthering their elected thought leader's academic career. This insidious yet incredibly powerful method—what amounts to a Trojan Horse of drug peddling—represents a betrayal of the average doctor seeing patients. (Lembke, 2016, p. 58–59)

Big Pharma has influenced pain doctors at academic conferences, and the doctors at the conferences were not made aware of the financial arrangements between the drug companies and the thought leader presentations (Lembke, 2016). Doctors rely on their colleagues to provide them with unbiased research at conferences.

Big Pharma has successfully framed opioids as the best way to manage pain without fully disclosing its funding for the research and researchers (Lembke, 2016). Goffman writes that "observers actively project their frames of reference on the world immediately around them" (p. 39); this frame analysis allows people to make assumptions about what is going on. Therefore, the world immediately around the doctors who attended the thought leader presentations projected their frames of pro-opioid prescribing (Lembke, 2016).

When analyzing framing, it is important to examine not only what is included in the frame but also what is excluded (Fairhurst and Sarr, 1996). Several studies indicate that opioids are appropriate for acute (short-term) pain but are not appropriate for chronic (long-term) pain (Chou, 2015). In terms of treatment for chronic pain, "evidence supports a dose-dependent risk for serious harms" (Chou, 2015, p. 276). Chou and his colleagues suggest that there is significant harm in long-term opioid usage, including increases in cardiovascular events, such as myocardial infarctions; the likelihood of fracture in the wrist, hip, and the humerus; and endocrinological harm (Chou, 2015, p. 278). Likewise, research suggests that "prescribing yet more imaging, opioids, injections, and operations is not likely to improve outcomes for patients with chronic back pain" (Deyo, 2009, p. 65). These and other studies have been excluded from the frame designed to cure the construct of *opiophobia.*

4.6 SOCIAL CONSTRUCTION, LANGUAGE, FRAMING, AND THE OPIOID CRISIS

Berger and Luckmann (1966) assert that reality is socially constructed and shaped by language. In essence, language gives legitimation to action, and it allows one to justify and explain actions (Berger and Luckmann, 1966, p. 64). Hence, it is worthy to explore the language employed in the episodic shift in the medical profession from conservative prescribing of opioids in the 1980s to liberal prescribing of opioids in the 1990s and 2000s (Lembke, 2016, p. 56).

Framing and language together can shape how others experience and interpret reality (Fairhurst and Sarr, 1996, p. X). Language is relevant to understanding the interpretative frame constructed. Fairhurst and Sarr (1996) illustrate, "Just as an artist works from a palette of colors to paint a picture, the leader who manages meaning works from a vocabulary of words and symbols to help construct a frame in the mind of the listener" (p. 100). The social construction of "opiophobia" convinced doctors that they had a fear of prescribing medicine to help patients feel relief (Lembke, 2016, p. 58). Additionally, the institution of the American Academy of Pain Management held some power and prestige. The American Academy of Pain Management thus was able to convey legitimacy in their rhetoric via thought leaders to create the perception that doctors had a disease to be cured, but the liberal prescribing of opioids has caused a spiraling out of control, leading to opioid addictions (Lembke, 2016). According to Berger and Luckmann (1966), "Theoretically sophisticated legitimations appear at particular moments of an institutional history," and the institutional history of the American Pain Society arguably was engaging in a paradigmatic shift in favor of opioid prescribing, relying heavily on thought leaders to encourage this shift (p. 65).

Thought leaders were instrumental in framing the pro-opioid stance (Catan and Perez, 2012; Lembke, 2016). One of the foremost thought leaders was Dr. Russell Portenoy (Lembke, 2016). Portenoy, a pain specialist at Beth Israel Medical Center in New York, championed the use of opioids for chronic pain in the 1990s (Catan and Perez, 2012). Purdue Pharma released videos featuring Portenoy and others citing the useful effects of opioids for relieving chronic pain. In these videos, Portenoy claimed that fewer than 1% of people who were prescribed these drugs would become addicted and that overdoses were rare (Catan and Perez, 2012). The catch phrase "fewer than 1% of people who are prescribed these drugs become addicted" appears frequently in the promotional materials. Such *catch phrases*, Fairhurst and Sarr (1996) explain, are helpful for framing a particular issue (p. 129).

Purdue Pharma frame opioids in a positive light with promotional videos and commercials that employ a *spin* to cast the subject (e.g., opioids) in a positive light (Fairhurst and Sarr, 1996, p. 101). For example, the Purdue Pharma OxyContin commercial entitled "I Got My Life Back," which aired in 1998, featured Dr. Alan Spanos stating,

> There's no question that our best and strongest pain medicines are the opioids, but these are the same drugs that have a reputation for causing addiction and other terrible things. Now in fact the rate of addiction amongst pain patients who are treated by doctors are less than 1%, they don't wear out, they go on working, they don't have serious medical side effects, and these drugs, I repeat, are our best, strongest pain medications and should be used much more than they are for patients in pain. (Spanos in *Purdue Pharma OxyContin Commercial*, 2016)

Narratives are powerful tools for framing: "Stories frame a subject by example and engage our attention and emotions. They are also useful teaching tools. Like metaphors, they can mask or hide meaning" (Fairhurst and Sarr, 1996, p. 129). Portenoy was persuasive because he successfully constructed a narrative to put doctors at ease and urge them to believe that prescribing opioids for chronic pain was best. In a 2011 live taped interview series entitled "Long-term Opioid Therapy Reconsidered, Addiction is not Rare in Pain Patients," Portenoy admits there are issues with the narrative he constructed. Portenoy says,

> I gave so many lectures to primary care audiences in which the Porter and Jick article was just one piece of data that I would then cite. I would cite 6 to 7 maybe 10 different avenues of thought or evidence, none of which represents real evidence. And yet what I was trying to do was to create a narrative so that the primary care audience would look at this information in toto and feel more comfortable about opioids in a way they hadn't before. . . . Because the primary goal was to de-stigmatize, we often left evidence behind. (*Opioids for Chronic Pain*, 2011)

The Porter and Jick article Portenoy mentions was relied upon heavily as *evidence* that opioids were safe. The Porter and Jick article is "an 11-line letter printed in the *New England Journal of Medicine* in January 1980" that refutes the claim that using opioids to treat chronic pain is risky (Moghe, 2016, p. 1). In this letter, Jane Porter and Dr. Hershel Jick conclude after performing an analysis of approximately 11,000 people that "the development of addiction is rare in medical patients with no history of addiction" (Porter and Jick in Moghe, 2016, p. 1). About six years later in May of 1986, Porteney and Foley published a study in the journal *Pain* where they conclude "that opioid maintenance therapy can be a safe, salutary and more humane alternative to the options of surgery or no treatment in those patients with intractable non-malignant pain and no history of drug abuse" (p. 171). The Porter and Jick article, along with the Portney and Foley article, serves as a complex metaphor in the framing process. Fairhurst and Sarr (1996) write that "complex metaphors have many implied meanings and represent useful tools around which to build a vision. In using them, we must be careful that they not diverge too far from images that others might expect" (p. 129). The aforementioned articles were relied upon as a metaphor for a pro-opioid stance. Framing tools, such as metaphors, catch phrases, spin, and narrative stories (Fairhurst and Sarr, 1996, p. 101), were used to construct the message that opioids were an appropriate treatment for chronic pain.

4.7 PAIN AS THE FIFTH VITAL, PATIENT SATISFACTION, AND "WHAT IS IT THAT'S GOING ON IN HERE?"

Frame analysis begins by considering the very broad question, "What is it that's going on in here?" although that question can create a bias toward a unitary moment in time and may guide perspective to a unitary event (Goffman, 1974, p. 9). Understanding the opioid crisis in "strips" or isolated parts allows for certain pieces of information to be pinpointed in the hopes of answering the question of "what is it that's going on here?"

Goffman (1974) claims, "My aim is to try to isolate some of the basic frameworks of understanding available in our society for making sense out of events and to analyze the special vulnerabilities to which these frames of reference are subject" (Goffman, 1974, p. 10). One basic framework of understanding worth isolating is the social construct of pain as the fifth vital sign. Patients in pain usually require qualitative assessment of their experience of the phenomenon of pain, but some doctors had concerns that pain was not being properly addressed. Because of these concerns, "in 1995, the American Pain Society (APS) set out guidelines delineating that a first step in improving the treatment of pain is assessment and recording of patients' reports of pain" (American Pain Society Quality of Care Committee quoted in Mularski et al., 2006, p. 607). The idea of quantifying pain was further addressed in 1996 when James Campbell, MD, in the presidential address to the American Pain Society, stated that "vital signs are taken seriously. . . . If pain were assessed with the same zeal as other vital signs are, it would have a much better chance of being treated properly" (Campbell quoted in Mularski et al., 2006, p. 607). The quantification of pain and the recognition of pain as the fifth vital sign happened formally in 1999 when the Veterans Health Administration (VHA) instituted an initiative called "Pain as the Fifth Vital" and required medical nurses to ask patients to rate their pain on a numeric rating scale (NRS) from 0 (no pain) to 10 (intense pain) (Mularski et al., 2006, p. 607). Any mention of a pain score over four would trigger "a comprehensive pain evaluation," and opioids were often considered (Mularski et al., 2006, p. 607). Also, the Joint Commission on Accreditation of Healthcare Organizations, now called the Joint Commission (JCO), began to support the usage of an NRS for reporting pain (Morone and Weiner, 2013, p. 1729).

Because of the combined power and prestige of the VHA and the JCO, most all other hospitals and medical practices followed suit in using the NRS (Morone and Weiner, 2013, p. 1729). When the VHA and JCO began engaging in self-reported pain assessment through an NRS, they established legitimacy to the practice of measuring pain as a number, 0 to 10. Berger and Luckmann (1966) explain, "Such knowledge constitutes the motivating dynamics of institutionalized conduct. It defines the institutionalized areas of conduct and designates all situations falling within them. It defines and constructs the roles to be played in the context of the institutions in question" (Berger and Luckmann, 1966, p. 65). The knowledge an organization produces and packages for external stakeholders provides a basis for evaluation.

The power and prestige of the Joint Commission, the American Pain Society, and the Veterans Administration constructed the discourse of the dominant episteme. Foucault (1980) explains, "The episteme is the 'apparatus' which makes possible the separation, not of the true from the false, but of what may from what may not be characterized as scientific" (Foucault, 1980, p. 197). In the historical moment 1990–1999, the scientific episteme was pain was undertreated and overlooked, that it must change, and it must change quickly (Meldrum, 2016).

The nurse becomes the recorder of the pain, the patient is the arbiter and measurer of the sensation of the pain, and the doctor is the one to *make the pain go away*. The institutional conduct and the roles of the participants is socially constructed. Responding to a numeric value for a pain level triggers a response by doctors to "treat" the pain.

Morone and Weiner (2013) explain opioid prescriptions increased due in part to patients' expectation that doctors respond to their pain complaint (p. 1729). Also, "another likely cause for the increased prescription of opioids is that writing a prescription is efficient" (p. 1730). Doctors typically have a limited amount of time to spend per patient; this may be a contributing factor to the opioid crisis as it leads to pain being addressed as a one-dimensional construct ignoring social, psychological, and cultural factors (Morone and Weiner, 2013).

Another exacerbating factor in the overprescribing of opioids is the linking of patient satisfaction to physician and hospital reimbursement (Fiore, 2016, p. 1). The Centers for Medicare and Medicaid Services (CMS) and the JCO are being urged to "re-examine its Pain Management Standards—which once helped push the idea of pain as the 'fifth vital sign'—and Physicians for Responsible Opioid Prescribing asked CMS to strike patient satisfaction questions about pain from its reimbursement procedures" (Fiore, 2016, p. 1). Numerous doctors signed a letter encouraging the removal of questions that link the quality of care and pain management from the Consumer Assessment of Healthcare Providers and Systems (HCAHPS) Survey, which links reimbursement to patient satisfaction. The letter specifically asks for the removal of the following questions:

1. During this hospital stay, did you need medicine for pain?
2. During this hospital stay, how often was your pain well controlled?
3. During this hospital stay, how often did the hospital staff do everything they could to help you with your pain? (Physicians for Responsible Opioid Prescribing, 2016b).

These questions are constructed to suggest that the doctor could have controlled or should have controlled the pain better. Also, the third question is constructed to frame the idea that the doctor or the staff may have withheld something from the patient when, in fact, prescribing more opioids could do more harm (Chou, 2015).

The medical literature (Morone and Weiner, 2013; Chou, 2015; and Lembke, 2016) and the humanities literature (Morris, 1998; Catt, 2012; and Gadamer, 1996) tend to agree with one another that pain is a multidimensional construct; cultural, social, biological, physiological, and psychological elements make up the *experience* of pain. The increase in the prescription of opioids "underscores the mistaken view that pain is a unidimensional problem" (Morone and Weiner, 2013, p. 1730). According to Morone and Weiner (2013), "When both patients and clinicians view pain as a purely sensory experience then management is necessarily limited to the sensation (and the prescription of pain medications). This approach is likely to result in a suboptimal patient response, especially when managing chronic pain" (p. 1730). Gadamer (1996) notes that health cannot only be treated "solely from the perspective of science" (p. viii). Hence, treating the mind, the body, and connection between the two may permit medical professionals to move closer to an optimal patient response.

4.8 CONCLUSIONS

There are limits to measurement, which, in Gadamer's (1996) opinion, "merits strong hermeneutical interest" (p. vii). Gadamer (1996) makes the point that modern science's goal of objectification and constant measurement is a "violent estrangement from ourselves" (p. 70). The idea that every patient in a medical setting must be evaluated via a numeric rating scale creates the idea that physical pain can be self-assessed on a sliding scale from 0–10. This notion seems to suggest a "violent estrangement" from one's being, as if one could separate mental pain from physical pain. The organization Physicians for Responsible Opioid Prescribing (PFROP) describe pain as a symptom of a larger issue, not merely a vital sign. In their letter to the JCO, members of PFROP write,

> Pain is a symptom, not a vital sign. Blood pressure, heart rate, respiratory rate and temperature are vital signs that can be objectively measured. Pain is only one of many distressing symptoms that patients can experience and to which health care professionals must be attentive. Pain is also not a single entity that warrants a formulaic "titrate to effect" approach in response to a patient's reported pain score. Mandating routine pain assessments for all patients in all settings is unwarranted and can lead to overtreatment and overuse of opioid analgesics. (2016a)

Regarding professional behavior, it is important to remember, "changing language can change behavior" (Kimball, 1996, p. 15). The language of *opiophobia* led physicians to believe that something was wrong within the physician community, and the idea that doctors needed to be cured of a socially constructed phobia led to overprescribing behaviors. When they heard thought leader presentations at medical conferences, doctors unknowingly were listening to presentations fully funded by Purdue Pharma, and they took the thought leader ideas back to their own praxis (Lembke, 2016). Patients suffering from chronic pain were initially enthused with opioids, thinking their pain would soon cease. One patient reports, "The doctor trusts me. He's also given me back my self-esteem and the ability to control myself. I'm empowered" (Meldrum, 2016, p. 1365). The sense of empowerment soon left and was replaced by lack of control and addiction (Meldrum, 2016, p. 1365). Language creates reality (Berger and Luckmann, 1966). The doctors' reality changed after hearing the rhetoric of Purdue Pharma, and doctors who blindly followed the rhetoric changed patients into opioid addicts who demanded more opioids.

Chapter Five

Human Flourishing

5.1 INTRODUCTION

This chapter looks to the literature of Aristotle about human happiness, the human need for the other, and contributions to the polis. This chapter asks what is the "good life?" How does human flourishing relate to the construct of pain? I plan to explore Arendt's *Human Condition* (2013) and her ideas about work, labor, and action and the rise of the social to the addiction crisis. Viktor Frankl's work on meaning and suffering is also applicable in this chapter. Frankl's (2011) insights are additive regarding ethics as his work *The Unheard Cry for Meaning* discusses ethics grounded in thoughtful action. Frankl, a survivor of concentration camps in Nazi Germany, writes about *crabbing*, a phenomenon in flying single-engine and twin-engine aircraft. In short, crabbing is when wind blows small planes away from their intended destination if their pilots are not cognizant of the direction of the wind; hence, pilots must be constantly aware of their path and *rechart* the course when needed to arrive at the correct destination. Frankl's crabbing metaphor insists that for awareness of thoughtful action, the actor must know the direction of the actions. Additionally, Frankl (1985) writes in the text *Man's Search for Meaning* that people act ethically not because they commit themselves to some great ethical cause but rather for the particular; therefore, according to Frankl, people act ethically because of love for another person or love for G-d. This chapter argues that the construct of Arendt's and Frankl's human flourishing may help those suffering from opioid addiction by providing an alternative to addiction and choose to live their life for the love of the other and serving the other. Frankl's studies suggest most people want to find their purpose and build a meaningful life.

I conclude the chapter asking, "Where do we go from here?" Medication-assisted treatment (i.e., Suboxone and methadone) would be appropriate to explore as it has been framed as a successful treatment and solution. Is medication-assisted treatment truly successful, or do reports of its success reflect still more branding that obfuscates the situation and simply transforms illegal addiction into corporate and state-sponsored addiction? This chapter acknowledges that there may never be an end to the opioid crisis rather there may simply be a lessening in the severity of the opioid crisis.

5.2 PHILOSOPHICAL CONNECTIONS TO HUMAN FLOURISHING

Happiness, or, as Aristotle says, "eudaimonia," is not a fleeting moment of enjoyment; by "eudaimonia," Aristotle is referring to "a life that is most desirable and satisfying" (Ross, 2009, p. xxvii). In antiquity, Aristotle (2011a) outlines what does not constitute happiness and the types of lives that should be avoided when trying to achieve a fulfilled and happy life (1.5–1.7). He explains that a life of pleasure-seeking is not for people but for hedonist "beasts," and people should avoid a life of simple hedonistic pursuits (2011a, 1.5). Aristotle (2011a) suggests avoiding a life of politics; such a life does not lead to happiness because the political life is too often focused on the politician rather than on the polis members. He explains the focus of a political life is on "those who bestow honor rather than on him who receives it" (2011a, 1.5). For the sake of happiness, one should also avoid a life focused only on making money. Aristotle concludes making money is a "compulsion" and that money is only "useful for the sake of something else," that there is no end attached to it (2011a, 1.6). A life focused only on the accumulation of money and material possessions does not move a person closer to eudaimonia.

To achieve eudaimonia, one must be an active participant in life; eudaimonia is an active pursuit because "human good turns out to be the soul exhibiting excellence" (Aristotle, 2011a, 1.7). Aristotle (2011a) provides the example of a lyre player and a good lyre player, concluding that the lyre player who plays well is moving toward eudaimonia. Living a connected life by participating and contributing to the polis is an essential part of "the good life," too, as "man was born for citizenship" (1.7). Another component of a life marked with eudaimonia is contemplation. With contemplation comes the ability to have the time to think, read, and learn.

Hannah Arendt's (1963; 2013) work describes what it means for a life to be whole and for humans to flourish. Arendt, like Aristotle, writes about contribution to the polis, action, and contemplation. Labor, work, and action are inescapable. Labor, as she defines it, is "the activity which corresponds to the biological process of the human body, whose spontaneous growth, metabolism, and eventual decay are bound to the vital necessities produced and fed into the life process by labor" (Arendt, 2013, p. 7). In Arendtian terms, this definition of labor includes the tasks that must be completed to make way for work to occur. Work, therefore, is worldliness; "Work provides an artificial world of things, distinctly different from all natural surroundings" (Arendt, 2013, p. 7). Work contributes to the polis through the production of goods and services. Last, and perhaps most important, is the concept of action, which involves the public and open discourse. Arendt writes, "Action, the only activity that goes on directly between men without the intermediary of things or matter, corresponds to the human condition of plurality, to the fact that men, not Man, live on Earth and inhabit the world" (Arendt, 2013, p. 7). Arendt explains that, in the time of the Roman empire, the terms "to live" and "to be among men" were synonymous (Arendt, 2013, p. 8). People need people for action, and, despite human similarities, no one's lived experience is identical to another. The concept of many participating, making their ideas known to other "men," is another part of action. All three categories—labor, work, and action—have a symbiotic relationship and "are intimately connected with the most general condition of human existence; birth and death, natality and mortality" (Arendt, 2013, p. 9). Labor, in its most basic form, ensures people can survive; work allows for human artifacts; and action preserves political bodies.

In Arendt's (2013) work the human condition is "not the same as the sum of total human activity"; the human condition encompasses more, such as the ability for contemplation (p. 10). The search for understanding of the human condition turns to the ability of men to think and contemplate ideas. With a life full of action (*activa*) to meet the needs of everyday life, the only way a person can move toward eudaimonia is to have both the time and the ability to contemplate ideas. *Vita completiva* ("life of contemplation") fits Arendt's rhetorical theory: People need to think for themselves and have the capacity to understand how *vita activa* ("action") will have consequences in society.

One of the major figures Arendt (1963) writes about is Adolf Eichmann, a Nazi who killed many. Eichmann's defense was he was merely following orders (Arendt, 1963, p. 1–10). Eichmann's actions and lack of contemplation illustrate that action without thought is dangerous. Arendt further explains the ability to contemplate and think: "However monstrous the deeds were, the doer was neither monstrous nor demonic, and the only specific characteristic one could detect in his past as well as in his behavior during the trial and the preceding police examination was something entirely negative; it was not stupidity but a curious, quite authentic inability to think" (Arendt, 1971, p. 417). The ability to combine contemplation and action is imperative for considering the implications of one's actions.

The *vita activa* gives rise to the Aristotelian concept of the "good life," which is "good . . . by having mastered the necessities of sheer life, by being freed from labor and work" (Arendt, 2013, p. 37). In *The Human Condition*, it becomes clear that, to Arendt, rhetoric is the marriage of action and rhetoric located only inside the polis with the presence of other people. The polis, the community or society in which one lives, is vital because "all human activities are conditioned by the fact that men live together, but it is only action that cannot even be imagined outside the society of men" (Arendt, 2013, p. 22). As noted previously, work and labor have their roles in a society, but a polis cannot exist without action. Action alone is the "exclusive prerogative of man," and man, according to Aristotle, is a political animal (Arendt, 2013, p. 23). The rise of the city-state in ancient Greece gave rise to a second life, a public life. A public life, or what Aristotle called a "bios politikos," consisted of two main parts: action (*praxis*) and speech (*lexis*). The belief that praxis and lexis capacities belong together is not original to Arendt. She explains these ideas in context with the stature of the Homeric Achilles, writing, "The stature of the Homeric Achilles can be understood only if one sees him 'as the doer of great deeds and the speaker of great words'" (Arendt, 2013, p. 25). This relationship between praxis and lexis, action and rhetoric, is the heartbeat of the vita activa: "To be political, to live in a polis, meant that everything was decided through words and not through force and violence" (Arendt, 2013, p. 26). This is the essence of the action-rhetoric relationship and serves as a coordinate to locate Arendt's work within the broader scope of rhetorical tradition. Lastly, Arendt's and Aristotle's works stress the need for participation in the polis. To be situated in the polis allows for the conditions necessary for human flourishing to occur.

5.3 MEANING IN LIFE

Viktor Frankl was an extraordinary man, a medical doctor and therapist who survived the Nazi concentration camps in Auschwitz, Poland (Redsand, 2006). Frankl was trained as a doctor specializing in both psychiatry and neurology. He organized suicide-prevention centers for teenagers in his hometown of Vienna, Austria, and his work with suicidal people led him to develop logotherapy. A main component of logotherapy was "that finding meaning in life can enable a person to survive the worst conditions" (Redsand, 2006, p. 4). Frankl's ideas about logotherapy occurred prior to his detention in the concentration camps, as he writes about having a manuscript tucked inside his coat when he arrived at the camp. From the following account, it is clear that Frankl's (1985) work was important to him:

> I tried to take one of the old prisoners into my confidence. Approaching him furtively, I pointed to the roll of paper in the inner pocket of my coat and said, "Look, this is the manuscript of a scientific book. I know what you will say; that I should be grateful to escape with my life, that that should be all I can expect of fate. But I cannot help myself. I must keep this manuscript at all costs; it contains my life's work. Do you understand that? (p. 13)

The idea that Frankl maintained the importance of his work to himself at the moment of such agony in a Nazi death camp is a realization that Frankl lived his life for the other. The nature of logotherapy, Frankl's work, helps the other who is in distress by helping the other see meaning in both life and suffering. Frankl writes, "A literal translation of the term 'logotherapy' is 'therapy through meaning.' Of course, it could also be translated as 'healing through meaning,' although this would bring in a religious overtone that is not necessarily present in logotherapy. In any case, logotherapy is a meaning-centered (psycho-) therapy" (Frankl, 2011, p. 1). Frankl's (1985) work, writings, and lived experience encourage anchoring one in one's life with the other and grounding one's existence in a life of thoughtful action (p. 37–45). Frankl (1985) cites a French study in which 89% of people asserted that a person needs "something" to live for, and Frankl completes his own study by asking people similar questions, yielding similar results (p. 100). Frankl (1985) also cites a study from Johns Hopkins University in which 78% of those surveyed considered "finding a purpose and meaning to [their] life" as a primary goal (p. 100).

It is the loved one in the background or the love of G-d in the background that foregrounds and shapes action; for example, Frankl's love for his wife gave his life meaning. As he marched in the snow and ice as a frail, malnourished prisoner, Frankl mentally clung to the image of his wife, and the love and admiration he had for her fueled him at his weakest moments (Frankl, 1985, p. 102). Frankl (1985) writes:

> A thought transfixed me: for the first time in my life I saw the truth as it is set into song by so many poets, proclaimed as the final wisdom by so many thinkers. The truth—that love is the ultimate and the highest goal to which man can aspire. Then I grasped the meaning of the greatest secret that human poetry and human thought and belief have to impart: The salvation of man is through love and in love. I understood how a man who has nothing left in this world still may know bliss, be it only for a brief moment, in the contemplation of his beloved. (p. 37)

The love of the other is the background that serves as a guiding principal in action.

Frankl is clear—Love is not a fleeting, momentary feeling; rather, love for the other is seen through action. One's active life involves intentionality and planning; Frankl illustrates this through the metaphor of crabbing. In a single-engine airplane, if the pilot does not plan for the winds correctly, the airplane will go askew. The pilot must have a destination in mind to arrive there successfully. Frankl (2011) gives this example:

> Let me here repeat an illustration that has often shown to be didactically helpful. In aviation there is a business called "crabbing." Say there is a crosswind from the north and the airport where I wish to land lies due east. If I fly east, I will miss my destination because my plane will have drifted to the southeast. In order to reach my destination, I must compensate for this drift by crabbing, in this case by heading my plane in a direction to the north of where I want to land. It is similar with man: he too ends at a point lower than he might have unless he is seen on a higher level that includes his higher aspirations. (p. 257–261).

Likewise, people "drift" away from a whole life without a clear understanding of their intended destination.

5.4 PHILOSOPHICAL CONNECTIONS

Aristotle, Arendt, and Frankl contribute valuable insights regarding how people can live the "good life," and many of their ideas can be put into conversation with one another. Aristotle, Arendt, and Frankl all recognize the importance of meaningful contribution to the polis. Frankl's (1985; 2011) work instructs readers to live for the other and that enduring suffering and emotional and physical pain is worthwhile because of the love of the other (1985, p. 37; 2011, p. 1). Also, Frankl's (1985) lived experience and the lengths he went to protect his manuscript illustrate the value of a professional life whereby one is contributing to the polis (1985, p. 3). Frankl (2011), like Aristotle, explains life cannot be just about making money:

> Today, to be sure, we also have to cope with unintentional leisure in the form of unemployment. Unemployment may cause a specific neurosis—"unemployment neurosis," as I called it when I first described it in 1933. But again, upon closer investigation it turned out that the real cause was the confusion of one's being unemployed with his being useless and, hence, his life's being meaningless. Financial compensation, or for that matter social security, is not enough. Man does not live by welfare alone. (p. x)

Meaningful work is important to a whole life. Aristotle explains making money is a compulsion with no end. Thus, Frankl elaborates that meaningful work contributes to a flourishing existence.

Aristotle warns against the dangers of isolation. He explains self-sufficiency is not the same as man not needing one another. Man is born for citizenship; hence, man needs man to reach his highest potential, and each polis should contribute (Aristotle, 2011a). Aristotle champions the importance of the polis and the other and their role in the good life. Frankl goes so far as to say the other is everything to live for and that, without the other, one may lose the will to carry on: "If a person has found the meaning sought for, he is prepared to suffer, to offer sacrifices, even, if need be, to give his life for the sake of it. Contrariwise, if there is no meaning he is inclined to take his life, and he is prepared to do so even if all his needs, to all appearances, have been satisfied" (Frankl, 2011, 129–130). The other gives reason to carry on in the face of great pain.

The *vita activa*, on which Arendt (2013), too, agrees with Aristotle, is a vital part of a whole life. Arendt emphasizes the relationship between people and lexis and praxis (p. 25). Arendt (2013) writes, "No other human performance requires speech to the same extent as action" (p. 179). So, to achieve true action and to contribute to the plurality of the political arena, people need a community of others who also participate. To Arendt, speech reveals the "unique identity of the person," and people "insert [themselves] in the world through speech and action" (Sarin, 2009, p. 99). People make sense of their existence to others and to themselves through speech. People "can experience meaningfulness only because they can talk with and make sense to each other and to themselves" (Arendt, 2013, p. 4). The importance of speech reveals the importance of the other in Arendt's work.

5.5 THE FUTURE INSTITUTION

Human flourishing and focusing on the other are key components for moving toward a life filled with eudaimonia. Moreover, human flourishing and focusing on the other are key components in an active and contemplative life. But these elements are not present when one is plagued with addiction. Living for the other is nearly impossible when one is gripped with addiction. Life becomes marked with dysfunction because "addiction is defined as a chronic relapsing brain disease that is characterized by compulsive drug seeking and use despite harmful consequences" (National Institute on Drug Abuse, 2014, p. 1). In the current historical moment, America is clearly amid an opioid addiction crisis; "From 2000 to 2014, nearly half a million persons in the United States have died from drug overdoses. In 2014, there [were] approximately one and a half times more drug overdose deaths in the United States than deaths from motor vehicle crashes" (Rudd et al., 2016, p. 1234). Opioids and heroin are the main drugs associated with overdose deaths (Rudd et al., 2016, p. 1234).

Chapter 4 established an institutional connection to the opioid crisis. Some argue the institutional change at the Veterans Hospitals was a contributing factor to the opioid crisis (Physicians for Responsible Opioid Prescribing, 2016a). Pain became recognized as the fifth vital sign, so major intuitions like the Veterans Hospital began implementing a numeric rating scale for the sensation of pain. In the early 1990s, many physicians argued pain was not being taken seriously. In response to their concerns, "in 1995, the American Pain Society (APS) set out guidelines delineating that a first step in improving the treatment of pain is assessment and recording of patients' reports of pain" (APS Quality of Care Committee in Mularski et al., 2006, p. 607). Furthermore, in the 1996 presidential address to the APS, James Campbell, MD, stated that "vital signs are taken seriously. . . . If pain were assessed with the same zeal as other vital signs are, it would have a much better chance of being treated properly" (Mularski et al., 2006, p. 607). The quantification of pain and the recognition of pain as the fifth vital sign happened formally in 1999 when the Veterans Health Administration (VHA) instituted an initiative called "Pain as the Fifth Vital" which required medical nurses to ask patients to rate their pain on a numeric rating scale (NRS) from 0 (no pain) to 10 (intense pain) (Mularski et al., 2006, p. 607). Both Arendt and Frankl stress the need for contributing to the polis through meaningful work, discourse, and connections to other. This section explores Jesse Brown Veterans Hospital, and it seems that their newest program to reduce pain aligns with Frankl's and Arendt's assertions.

How can institutions undo the damage of overprescribing opioids for chronic pain? The answer may be nuanced, but the Jesse Brown Veterans Hospital in Chicago is trying innovative programs that allow relief for those suffering from chronic pain, but not through opioids. One hundred and three veterans with chronic pain at the Jesse Brown Veterans Hospital attended a "Pain Education School," and these participants have demonstrated "promising scientific evidence to support their use for chronic noncancer pain conditions" (Cosio and Lin, 2015, p. 1). Specific options listed in the study's conclusion are "acupuncture, biofeedback/relaxation training, movement (yoga), and spinal manipulation" (Cosio and Lin, 2015, p. 1). The Pain Education School taught patients about complementary and alternative medicine (CAM) options. Pain Education School covers topics such as "Acceptance & Commitment Therapy/mindfulness, acupuncture, aromatherapy, biofeedback/relaxation training, chiropractor, healing touch, hypnosis, massage, movement (e.g., yoga), music/art therapy, spinal manipulation, spirituality/religion, and traditional healers" (Cosio and Lin, 2015, p. 1). The study distinguishes between active, passive, and transitional CAM options. Active CAM options are movement programs, music therapy, art therapy, and mindfulness training; passive CAM options include acupuncture and massage therapy (Bender, 2017). Transitional CAM options are chiropractic care and osteopathic manipulation (Bender, 2017). The results of the current study confirm that there was a paradigm shift among the patients to using CAM modalities upon completion of the pain education program because the veteran is made aware of the CAM options and the benefits associated (Cosio and Lin, 2015, p. 1). Thus, the study has two major findings: "At most, providers may want to begin practicing 'integrative' medicine," and, at the very least, "doctors must address 'lifestyle imbalances' affected by chronic pain, including stress, physical activity, sleep, and nutrition, and make appropriate recommendations and referrals" (Cosio and Lin, 2015, p. 1). The idea of relying on complementary and alternative medicine to treat pain is a paradigmatic shift away from pharmacological options.

Another innovative program took place at Jesse Brown VA Medical Center and was implemented mainly by David Cosio, PhD, Psychologist; Dr. Schaefer; and dietitian Shari Pollack. Cosio et al. (2017) created functional medicine teams:

> [Fifty-one] Veterans aged 18–75 years old with chronic pain conditions were recruited for a pilot Functional Medicine clinic at Jesse Brown VA Medical Center between May 4, 2016–April 26, 2017. The group treatment protocol consist[ed] of four sessions that were approximately 60–75 minutes in duration. Patients were coached to change their environment and live an anti-inflammatory lifestyle. (2017, p. 1)

The purpose of the study was to "determine whether participation in the Functional Medicine clinic would significantly decrease pain intensity, weight, waist/hip circumference, medical symptoms/toxicity, perceived stress, insomnia, and increase walking speed" (Cosio et al., 2017, p. 1). Veterans who participated in the functional medicine clinic experienced a "decreased stress level and a decrease in joint and muscle symptoms" (Cosio et al., 2017, p. 1). These innovative programs encourage being an active and thoughtful participant in one's life; both of the aforementioned studies emphasize active modalities such as exercise, yoga, deep breathing, and meditation. Additionally, the emphasis on mindfulness, changes in diet, and changes to thought processes cannot be ignored when considering alternatives to pain management.

A few small-scale studies are encouraging, but institutions cannot end the opioid crisis alone; doctors are the first responders to pain and must engage in a paradigmatic shift away from overprescribing opioids and addiction.

5.6 PARADIGM SHIFTS IN MEDICINE TO ADDRESS THE OPIOID CRISIS

Regarding the shift needed to address the opioid crisis, Lembke (2016) summarizes the issue best, "Medicine must once and for all embrace addiction as a disease, not because science argues for it, but because it is practical to do so" (Lembke, 2016, p. 153). Sturgeon and Zautra (2016) report "social factors may increase vulnerability to chronic pain via both focal exposure to major life stressors (e.g., trauma) and through chronic exposure to socially painful situations (e.g., ostracism, isolation, and prolonged social conflict)" (p. 63). However, the medical system may be contributing to the problem because the medical system tends to "ostracize patients with addiction, especially while openly embracing and aggressively treating disorders such as chronic pain, chronic fatigue, fibromyalgia, depression, attention deficit disorder, and so on" (Lembke, 2016, p. 153). Patients suffering from the aforementioned diseases are overprescribed prescription medicines. As long as people are overprescribed medicines, the drug epidemic will continue, and so will the suffering of millions of people with untreated addiction (Lembke, 2016).

Lembke (2016) explains that the average doctor lacks knowledge in addiction because addiction education is mostly nonexistent from almost all medical school's curriculum and residency training programs, including many psychiatry residencies (Lembke, 2016). There is a new subspecialty of medicine called "addiction medicine," but, at present "insufficient access to treatment is a function of relatively low levels of professional experts in addiction medicine" (Rasyidi et al., 2012, p. 461). Other factors must also be addressed beyond the shortage of doctors trained in addiction medicine. Lembke (2016) provides an example of Susie who is an addiction medicine doctor, and her employment situation makes her quite precarious. Susie does not receive a base salary, nor does she receive health insurance or a retirement package. "Whether I spend a lot of time or a little time with one patient," Susie said, "I get paid only for what I bill. If the crux of my interaction with patients is a conversation, I lose dollars, because talking doesn't pay" (Susie in Lembke, 2016, p. 121). Addiction medicine is not respected in terms of salary or time spent per patient, and financial considerations may be driving many issues in overprescribing (Lembke, 2016, p. 133).

Aristotle in 333 BCE understood the dangers of focusing on moneymaking as it becomes a compulsion without an end, and this danger is still relevant in a twenty-first-century clinical setting (2011a, p. 1.7). Lembke (2016) explains doctors are pressured to see several patients to make money for the hospital system. "Addiction treatment must be delivered in a chronic-care model that prioritizes the importance of the doctor-patient relationship and the therapeutic environment" (p. 153). Patients must have the time with their doctor to talk and not feel rushed. Making the time to listen is a "precursor for empathic listening, informed judgment, and the healing power of human connection" (Lembke, 2016, p. 153). Time spent with patients tends to lead to better outcomes. "When patients get more time with doctors, they tend to be more satisfied with their care, experience reduced rates of medication prescriptions, and be less likely to file malpractice claims" (Franklin, 2021, para 10). But time is too often in short supply.

Lembke (2016) provides a specific example which homes in on the moneymaking compulsion. Psychiatrists offer a service called "medication management." Medication management does not focus on talk therapy and only a few minutes are spent with each patient. The psychiatrist can bill a minimum of $230 for this service, and the brevity of the appointment allows for many more patients per unit time. "It is no wonder, then, that a whole generation of psychiatrists now calls themselves 'psychopharmacologists,' doing nothing more than prescribing psychotropic drugs" (121).

Lembke (2016) then contrasts this moneymaking scenario with a 50-minute psychotherapy session that generates $300 and involves more time talking to the patient and addressing biosocial and cultural factors. Based on Lembke's figures, a psychiatrist could see six people for a total of ten minutes each, generating $230 x 6 people = $1,380, or the psychiatrist could talk to one person and generate $300. Most concerning is that "the pressure to see more patients per unit time and to bill more per patient pervades all of medicine, encouraging doctors to continue to prescribe drugs," thus becoming a vicious cycle of visiting a doctor to get rid of pain and only receiving a pill which may create an ongoing addiction (Lembke, 2016, p. 121).

5.7 PARADIGM SHIFT TO GETTING IT RIGHT

One program offered in Kaiser Permanente Hospital's Chronic Pain Management Department in San Francisco frames pain management through a nonpharmacological approach. The program's brochure explains, "Program participants learn a variety of nonpharmacologic pain management skills including physical, psychological, and psychophysiological coping skills that improve functioning and quality of life" (Mikeladze et al., n.d., p. 1). The overarching goals of the program are adequate pain control, reduction in suffering, the establishment of effective social support, and improved function

(Mikeladze et al., n.d., p. 1). The Kaiser program frames chronic pain as a construct with physical, emotional, and behavioral elements. The program services include pain education classes, family sessions, aftercare program with exercise, medication management, acupuncture, and biofeedback (Mikeladze et al., n.d., p. 1). Because "our culture—the modern, Western, industrial, technocratic world—has succeeded in persuading us that pain is simply and entirely a medical problem," the Kaiser program has responded by deconstructing this notion and addressing more than just the sensation of nerves (Morris, 1998). The Kaiser program strives for a holistic view of a person by increasing functioning (returning to meaningful work, mindfulness, active exercise), living for the other (social support and family classes), and active exercise.

In 2010, each Kaiser facility was encouraged to develop programs that address patient issues with chronic pain and addiction (Lembke, 2016, p. 154). As a result, Karen Peters, a clinical psychologist at Kaiser Santa Clara Chemical Dependency and Rehabilitation Program, and Barbara Gawehn, a registered nurse, developed a program to address the phenomena of prescription opioid abuse and addiction (Lembke, 2016, p. 154–158). Peters and Gawehn created a program that required initial daily visits to provide psychosocial support for patients in opioid withdrawal and struggling with pain without opioids. Peters and Gawehn's approach focused on building a supportive community and all psychotherapy and physical therapy was performed in groups, because building a supportive community between patients was at the heart of their approach.

Peters and Gawehn's program addresses the underlying issues with pain and relies upon changing the chronic pain narrative from pain being something that rules one's life to pain being something one handles. This program provides tools for patients to be in control of their pain. Peters and Gawehn's program commences every morning with "mindfulness meditation, chi gong, yoga, educational seminars, cognitive behavioral therapy, Feldenkrais, and even physical therapy" (Lembke, 2016, p. 155). These experiences, when performed as a group, "build a common language, one that serves to shape an illness narrative, the core of which is that they need to 'retrain their nervous system' to find a different way to manage pain." (Lembke, 2016, p. 155). The framing of pain in the narrative of the Kaiser program is one of patient empowerment and putting the patient in a place to develop skill sets to cope with pain. In this model, a chronic pain cure is not found in a quick-fix bottle of opioids.

The Kaiser Model, whereby complementary and alternative medicine (CAM) are the central focus of treatment, is in the minority as most programs treat opioid addiction pharmacologically. Of the millions of people who suffer from chronic pain and opioid addiction, "Fewer than 200,000 patients currently participate in multidisciplinary treatment" (Meldrum, 2016, p. 1365). The reason for the small number of patients who participating is attributed to the reluctance of insurers to cover costly programs (Meldrum, 2016, p. 1365).

Buprenorphine, which is sold under the branded names Suboxone®, Subutex®, Zubsolv®, Bunavail™, and Probuphine®, is an opioid medication used to treat opioid addiction (U.S. Food and Drug Administration in NAABT, 2018, p. 1). According to the National Alliance of Advocates for Buprenorphine Treatment,

> Buprenorphine is an opioid, and thus can produce typical opioid effects and side effects such as euphoria and respiratory depression, its maximal effects are less than those of full agonists like heroin and methadone. At low doses Buprenorphine produces sufficient agonist effect to enable opioid-addicted individuals to discontinue the misuse of opioids without experiencing withdrawal symptoms. The agonist effects of Buprenorphine increase linearly with increasing doses of the drug until it reaches a plateau and no longer continues to increase with further increases in dosage. This is called the "ceiling effect." Thus, Buprenorphine carries a lower risk of abuse, addiction, and side effects compared to full opioid agonists. In fact, Buprenorphine can actually block the effects of full opioid agonists and can precipitate withdrawal symptoms if administered to an opioid-addicted individual while a full agonist is in the bloodstream. (2018, p. 1)

A study published in 2007 from the *Journal of Addiction Medicine* reports,

> Suboxone is an effective intervention for treating opioid dependence that is amenable for use in multiple treatment settings, including solo primary care practices. In the present report, Suboxone maintenance reduced opioid use, was not associated with any serious adverse events, was associated with high rates of treatment retention and helped reach a broad patient population, especially those who had never before received opioid agonist medication-assisted therapy. (Finch et al., 2007, p. 104)

However, one is left questioning: If Suboxone and Subutex were approved by the FDA to treat opioid addiction in 2002, why are 129 people dying every day from opioid overdoses? (Kodjak, 2016, p. 1).

5.8 CONCLUSION

Human flourishing and moving toward full potential are virtually impossible in the tight grip of addiction as addiction robs the ability to create a life with eudaimonia at the center. When addicted and in chronic pain, patients often wait anxiously for their next dose of medicine. By that point, the pills do not relieve the pain; rather, the pills feed the opioid addiction (Lembke, 2016, p. 58–90). Frankl's (2011) work advises that the reason to live is found in the love for the other (*The Unheard Cry for Meaning*) and that, when life goes adrift, people must plan to pull their lives back together. Frankl's work accounts for humans making mistakes, learning, and recharting their life course. In fact, they must, for Frankl (2011) explains,

> Otherwise man will "drift," he will deteriorate, for there is a human potential at its worst as well. We must not let our belief in the potential humanness of man blind us to the fact that humane humans are and probably always will be a minority. Yet it is this very fact that challenges each of us to join the minority: things are bad, but unless we do our best to improve them, everything will become worse. (p. 29–30).

One must make the choice to act humane, to act from a place of love, and to strive to be better.

Arendt's (1963; 2013) work is also applicable when facing addiction to opioids, as her work calls for the value of meaningful action performed in conjunction with thoughtful contemplation. Arendt's work specifically calls patients to question and think before mindlessly following doctors' orders. Moreover, Arendt's work calls the professional—in this case, the doctor—not to partake mindlessly in a broken system where the evidence is lacking that connects diminished chronic pain with opioid usage (Arendt, 1963; 2013). Finally, Arendt's work encourages thoughtful consideration of complementary and alternative medicine treatments to address chronic pain.

Patients are dying every day from addiction; addiction now kills more people than car crashes each year (Lembke, 2016, p. 4). Chronic pain and addiction to opioids create an addictive cycle where one needs more opioids because of the underlying addiction. Addiction is a brain-based disease which must be addressed through biological, social, and cultural means (Morris, 1998, p. 1–10). Addressing chronic pain in a paradigm like the Kaiser programs and the Jesse Brown Veteran's Hospital are the key to helping people become free from the chaos addiction creates. Both Arendt and Frankl stress the need for contributing to the polis through meaningful work, the power of discourse, and connections to the other. The Kaiser programs and the Jesse Brown Veteran's Hospital incorporate many of these values as part of building a fulfilling and connected life free from addiction.

Chapter Six

Innocent Victims in the Opioid Crisis

The tiniest victims of this crisis are the newborn babies who are born drug-addicted and in pain by no fault of their own. This chapter explores the question "How is the opioid crisis impacting families and children?" The infant exposed to opioids in utero frequently presents a challenge in terms of development, eating, and self-soothing to doctors and caregivers (Jannson et al., 2009, p. 47). Considering the aforementioned challenges, how are the dangers of opioids being communicated to women in general and to pregnant mothers?

Health communication and the implications of campaigns to reach potential new mothers are of scholarly interest "as communication scholars [discuss] the importance of reflective thinking about the capacity of campaigns to effect change; this reflective thinking is especially important in the realm of the increasing gaps in society between the health rich and the health poor and the increasing marginalization of the poorer sections of society" (Dutta-Bergman, 2005, p. 103). Women—or pregnant mothers—should not be treated as a monolith population, and socioeconomic status impacts the likelihood of being prescribed an opioid. Many of the mothers who are prescribed opioids are on government-supplemented Medicaid; actually, "39% of Medicaid-enrolled women aged 15–44 years [filled a] prescription for an opioid medication each year for five consecutive years" (Ailes in Kraft, 2016, p. 203). Medicaid-enrolled pregnant women from 47 states in the United States reported that 21.6% of the women filled at least one opioid prescription during their pregnancy and this is higher than the 14.4% of women who were on private commercial insurance (Yazdy et al., 2015). In a cohort of more than 1 million Medicaid-enrolled pregnant women, about one in five women was dispensed prescription opioids during pregnancy and there was a substantial increase in filled prescriptions between 2000 and 2007 (Desai et al., 2014). This statistic caused me to question, are there any public health campaigns constructed to target potential new moms of all socioeconomic statuses and varying education levels? What may be some possible options to consider in terms of campaigns?

This chapter also considers the intersection of health communication and family communication. Women of color and pregnant mothers are disproportionately incarcerated and impacted by addiction than their white counterparts (Costa and Borrowman, 2004). Ritchie's (2017) *Invisible No More* works toward an understanding of policing and criminalization, exposing how women on the "margins" end up separated from their young children. There are vast implications to the family unit and communication patterns in times of crisis. Because parents and children form a familial bond, "families and how they communicate matter in health communication" (Pecchioni and Keeley, 2011, p. 353). The family unit is thought to provide supportive communication for one another. Moss (1973) defines the function of social support as it "provides each person with a communication network that is a safe base. Here [one] can be accepted whether he succeeds or fails in other networks. Here [one] can retreat to take stock of [himself/herself] and prepare to meet 'life.' Here [one] is accepted as a 'whole person,' and all his various qualities, roles, desires, and the like are of interest" (p. 236–237). Supportive communication has been recognized as a "necessary condition for the quality of life and for healthful living" (Albrecht and Goldsmith, 2003, p. 325). Supportive communication has shown a consistent positive effect on health. The impact of social support is comparable to other well-known risk factors such as smoking, blood pressure, blood lipids, obesity, and physical activity (House et al. in Albrecht and Goldsmith, 2003, p. 326). An intact family unit that is not plagued with addiction may be able to offer the supportive communication mentioned above. This is in stark contrast to many families with infants and young children that are being torn apart by dysfunction from the opioid epidemic. The foster care system is struggling to keep up with demand (Collier, 2018, p. 18). The opioid crisis is affecting the family unit in a negative way, and children are often placed with family members other than their parents or in foster care.

6.1 INTRODUCTION

In chapters 3, 4, and 5, the ideas of the individual who is suffering from chronic pain and turns to opioids for relief of pain are explored. Opioids are not appropriate for treating chronic pain; hence, the pain problem leads to a new problem of addiction (Lembke, 2016; Chou, 2015; Physicians for Responsible Opioid Prescribing, 2016a). This chapter sheds light upon a different entity affected by the crisis: children. The opioid crisis in the United

States is of extreme concern in neonatal units across the country; for instance, "in 2012 nearly 22,000 babies were born drug-dependent, one every 25 minutes, according to the most recent federal data" (Smith, 2017, p. 1). Pregnant women with a hospital delivery in the United States reported a fourfold increase in opioid use reported during pregnancy from 1999 to 2014 (Haight et al., 2018).

Babies born addicted to opioids behave differently from babies who are born without being exposed to drugs in utero. Babies who are exposed to drugs in utero "shake, sweat, vomit, and hold their bodies stiff as planks. They eat and sleep fitfully" (Smith, 2017, p. 1). As a society, we owe our most precious resource—our children, the future of this nation—a healthy and nurturing start. This chapter seeks to understand the parameters of this.

6.2 HISTORICAL MOMENT AND LANGUAGE

The understanding that opioids are not a new pharmacological substance provides historical understanding of the development of the opioid epidemic in this historical moment. Recall from chapter 1 that the first opium use dates to the ancient civilizations of Mesopotamia (~3400 BCE), but the first surviving records of opium addiction date from the end of the eighteenth century (Kocherlakota, 2014). Opiates have been abused "since at least 300 BC [when] Nepenthe (Greek 'free from sorrow') helped the hero of the *Odyssey*, but widespread opium smoking in China and the Near East has caused harm for centuries" (Kosten and Haile, 2014, p. 468e).

Of particular interest to this chapter is the history of women and opioid usage. In the nineteenth century, morphine and heroin addictions among women were recorded; however, in the nineteenth century, "infants were not thought to be affected because it was believed that morphine use among women was associated with sterility and a loss of sexual desire" (Merry in Kocherlakota, 2014, p. e547). The questioning of the *old paradigm* (Kuhn, 1970, p. 12) about opium and dangers to infants began in 1875 "after the first reported case in a neonate who manifested signs of opioid withdrawal at birth and was diagnosed with congenital morphinism (Courtwright in Kocherlakota, 2014, p. e547). Other babies were reported with similar symptoms; however, due to lack of treatment and understanding of a neonate suffering from withdrawal, most babies born addicted to opioids in the late 1800s and early 1900s died.

The family structure has suffered historically when opium addiction has been prevalent in society. Opium was destructive to the family unit in China in the early twentieth century. Slack (2001) reports on a newspaper article highlighting the *pernicious influence* opioids had on the family unit. A story from Shanghai's newspaper the *Xinwenbao,* entitled "Never Live with an Opium Smoker," appeared in 1927 and chronicled the plight of Wang Quanlin:

> Wang Quanlin was the proprietor of a foreign goods store. He and his wife, Wang Zhongshi, had been married for over seventeen years and had produced several sons and daughters together. However, Zhongshi became addicted to opium several years earlier. She no longer assisted her husband in the family store, but instead spent all day long reclining and smoking opium to the neglect of her household duties. Many times Quanlin admonished his wife to seek treatment but to no avail. Later, his fifteen-year-old son and ten-year-old daughter imitated their mother's behavior and became addicted to the pipe. Mr. Wang began taking more severe measures against his spouse, and eventually divorced her on the grounds she was endangering the children. (Slack, 2001, p. 46–47)

The idea that neonates suffer when opioids are introduced in utero is not a new phenomenon. In 1903, a correspondent going only by the initials O. D. reported in *Journal of American Medical Association* (JAMA) about a baby who, on the second day of life, began to scream and cry uncontrollably and, for two additional days, continued to cry; the baby then was treated with 0.5 mg of morphine every other day and was able to recover (Perlstein, 1947, p. 633). In 1964, methadone was introduced to treat addiction, and it, too, had adverse effects on neonates, and, in 2002, Buprenorphine was also introduced in the United States to treat addiction; similarly, Buprenorphine continues to have adverse effects on neonates (Kocherlakota, 2014, p. e547). In the current historical moment, the United States is amid a crisis as the incidence of babies exposed to opioids during pregnancy is at an all-time high: "From 2004 through 2013, the rate of NICU admissions for the neonatal abstinence syndrome increased from 7 cases per 1000 admissions to 27 cases per 1000 admissions" (Tolia et al., 2005, p. 2118). In a period of about nine years, the problem has increased to levels never before seen in recorded medical history. Babies are suffering because women of childbearing age are taking opioids; "approximately 28% of privately insured and 39% of Medicaid-enrolled women age 15–44 years [filled a] prescription for an opioid medication each year for five consecutive years" (Ailes in Kraft, 2016, p. 203). Every 25 minutes in the United States, a baby is born addicted to opioids and suffering from withdrawal (U.S. Department of Health and Human Services, 2015).

Morris (1991) helps to explain the connections between chronic pain, opioid addiction, and the historical moment. In this postmodern moment, Morris (1991) asserts, chronic pain is the illness of *our* time (p. 65). Morris (1991) writes, "Chronic pain, indeed, though far less visible than cancer or AIDS, certainly belongs among the characteristic maladies of our time" (p. 65). AIDS and cancer have physical manifestations—extreme weight loss, fragility, and extremely pale coloring—but those with chronic pain often appear physically "normal." Morris (1991) understands chronic pain needs to be addressed differently than other diseases of our time: "What AIDS, cancer, tuberculosis, leprosy, madness, and other representative illnesses share is a graphic power to seize the imagination. They not only threaten personal and public health but also, equally important, fill the world with disturbing new images of our vulnerability to disaster" (Morris, 1991, p. 66). Someone with chronic pain could appear to be physically healthy, so one may have addiction and still be able to conceal that from the world. However, chronic pain and addiction to opioids do create an image of vulnerability in neonates born to drug-addicted mothers (Smith, 2017, p. 1–3). Moreover, babies born suffering from neonatal abtinence syndrome (NAS) do not behave nor appear physically healthy. Perhaps images and video highlighting the suffering of neonates born with NAS would help to convey the severity of the problem to the public.

In this historical moment, more people are being treated with opioids because of their chronic pain, including pregnant women; therefore, neonates are suffering. Babies born to drug-addicted mothers are said to be suffering from NAS (U.S. Department of Health and Human Services, 2015). NAS occurs when a baby is born because "opioids pass readily from a pregnant woman's bloodstream through the placenta and across the fetal blood-brain barrier. When birth abruptly shuts down the flow of the drug, the baby's nervous system can trigger the agitating symptoms of withdrawal" (Smith, 2017, p. 2). Babies are not labeled as addicts, nor are they suffering from addiction:

> Experts don't consider it to be addiction, which, by definition, means a person persists in compulsive drug use despite terrible consequences. By the same logic, NAS is also a misnomer—abstaining, or just saying no, is different from experiencing the physical anguish of withdrawal. But medical experts have come to accept the NAS label because it's less fraught with stigma than words like addiction and withdrawal. (Smith, 2017, p. 2)

NAS is a socially constructed term (Berger and Luckmann, 1966) so that newborn babies are not attached to a negative stigma. The etymology of the word "stigma" is from the Greeks, who relied on strong visual aids designed to expose something unusual or bad about the moral status of the signified (Goffman, 1963, p. 1). Neonates suffering from NAS are treated with methadone; the babies often suffer in pain. Smith explains the fragility of the babies and their needs. Hospital units for drug-addicted babies need "dim lights and hushed conversations because the babies need calm and quiet" (Smith, 2017, p. 2). Also, babies born to drug-addicted moms may need methadone or other medication to relieve their symptoms. They are weaned from it over days or weeks (Smith, 2017). Having one's existence begin wrought with pain and suffering is heartbreaking, so the question becomes what to do about it.

6.3 COMMUNICATING MEDICAL RISKS

Communication of health messages typically has two components: knowledge of the information and behavioral change (Schiavo, 2013). When a woman walks into the doctor's office with chronic pain and is prescribed an opioid, she may not be told the possible effects to her and her baby, if she were to get pregnant. Pain Medicine News reports, "Women of reproductive age are commonly prescribed opioids, and prescribing rates are consistently higher among women on Medicaid than those who are privately insured" (Gallagher et al. in Holzman, 2018, p. 1). In addition, "opioids can act as folic acid antagonists when they are taken up to two months before conception" (Holzman, 2018, p. 1). In other words, opioids can block the body from naturally processing folic acid. This is a problem because folic acid is important for the developing fetus as it can prevent neural tube defects. Researchers explain, "Spina bifida and anencephaly are common and serious birth defects. Available evidence indicates that 0.4 mg per day of folic acid, one of the B vitamins, will reduce the number of cases of neural tube defects (NTDs)" (Houk et al., 1992, p. 1).

Women are not being told about the risks of opioids to their reproductive health. In a 2013–2016 study, Dr. Hebecca Norwick and Linda Morgan, PhD, MSN, RN, assistant professor in the School of Nursing at the California State University in Sacramento, analyzed the rate of effective preconception care among women of reproductive age at a community health center (Holzman, 2018). In the study:

> The cohort included 145 women of reproductive age; 47 of the women, who ranged in age from 23 to 44 years, were receiving opioid prescriptions on an ongoing basis, Dr. Norwick noted. Seventy-two percent of the women were on Medicaid, 19% had no insurance and only 1% had private insurance. According to Dr. Norwick, 43% of the women of reproductive age on prescribed opioids received effective preconception counseling. (Holzman, 2018, p. 1)

This leads one to conclude 67% of the women did not receive any or any effective preconception counseling. The Centers for Disease Control and Prevention released a Morbidity and Mortality Weekly Report in 2016 offering implications for public health practice:

> Pregnancy status, sexual activity, and contraceptive use should be ascertained by providers before prescribing opioid pain medications; for women with chronic pain, recommendations from CDC's opioid prescribing guideline should be followed. For women with other pain conditions who are pregnant or who are not using contraceptives, adherence to acute care setting, dental practice, and other clinical practice guidelines facilitated through clinical quality improvement strategies might result in increased prescribing and use of safer pain medications or nonpharmacologic treatments. (Gallagher et al., 2016, p. 1)

Women need doctors to fulfill the Hippocratic Oath and first do no harm. The doctor has both a professional and ethical responsibility to make certain their patient is fully informed of risks of taking an opioid. In a review article about counseling women about the risks opioids pose to a pregnancy found a concerning trend; if a woman was not planning a pregnancy, there tends to be discussion about contraception options not effects of opioids to a potential fetus; however, up to 86% of pregnancies are unintended in women who are abusing opioids (Heil in Brennan and Rayburn, 2012). Women who are not planning a pregnancy are not told of the risks of the opioids, rather only the women who are planning a pregnancy are counseled on the risks (Brennan and Rayburn, 2012, p. 623). Another concern is in the general population "more than half of pregnancies are unintended; therefore, many first-trimester exposures to opioids occur before pregnancy confirmation" (Brennan and Rayburn, 2012, p. 620). Therefore, it is reasonable to conclude that many women who receive opioid prescriptions are not advised and counseled about potential risks the opioids may cause to a fetus.

6.4 POLICY, RED TAPE, AND DRUG QUALIFICATION

In the United States, the Food and Drug Administration (FDA) exists in the hopes of regulating food and drugs to help keep the American public safe and informed on both the benefits and the risks of what they ingest or inject into their bodies. The risks and adverse effects of drugs are relevant when considering the link between opioid consumption, women of childbearing age, and pregnancy. According to the U.S. Department of Health and Human Services, "American consumers benefit from having access to the safest and most advanced pharmaceutical system in the world. The main consumer watchdog in this system is FDA's Center for Drug Evaluation and Research (CDER)" (U.S. Department of Health and Human Services, 2018, p. 1). The CDER is responsible for reviewing all the information that drug companies submit:

> Drug companies seeking to sell a drug in the United States must first test it. The company then sends CDER the evidence from these tests to prove the drug is safe and effective for its intended use. A team of CDER physicians, statisticians, chemists, pharmacologists, and other scientists reviews the company's data and proposed labeling. If this independent and unbiased review establishes that a drug's health benefits outweigh its known risks, the drug is approved for sale. The center doesn't actually test drugs itself, although it does conduct limited research in the areas of drug quality, safety, and effectiveness standards. (2018, p. 1)

After the CDER approves a drug, there is an evaluation of risk management, as "all drugs have risks" (U.S. Department of Health and Human Services, 2018, p. 1). During the risk-management evaluation, an FDA-approved drug label is written that clearly describes the drug's benefits and risks. However, further effort is sometimes needed to understand and manage risk, and this calls for a drug maker to implement a Risk Evaluation and Mitigation Strategy (REMS): "The Food and Drug Administration Amendments Act of 2007 gave the FDA the authority to require a Risk Evaluation and Mitigation Strategy (REMS) from manufacturers to ensure that the benefits of a drug or biological product outweigh its risks" (U.S. Department of Health and Human Services & U.S. Food and Drug Administration, n.d., p. 1). Hence, the FDA is the gatekeeper for the public, and the FDA has a responsibility to explain risks and benefits of medications to doctors, pharmacists, and the patients through written warnings that are received with the medications.

In October 2010, a REMS was approved for the drug isotretinoin, Isotretinoin, is commonly sold under the name Accutane, and it is a powerful drug used in the treatment of acne (Wysowski et al., 2002, p. 505). Accutane/isotretinoin carries significant risks to babies, if a mother were to get pregnant while using the medication:

> Accutane is an extremely dangerous teratogen: it can cause severe birth defects when taken during pregnancy. About one quarter of babies born who have been exposed to Accutane during gestation have major congenital deformities. Those babies born without major malformations frequently develop severe learning disabilities. A whole segment of Accutane babies do not even survive pregnancy: 40% are spontaneously miscarried. (Green, 2002, p. 1)

When women of childbearing age are prescribed Accutane, prescribers adhere to REMS materials to counsel them. A DVD is provided to all doctors wanting to prescribe the medication, and the script from the video makes the risks very clear to providers and patients alike. The video stresses all the negative effects to the unborn baby; for example,

- "One of these birth defects may be abnormal skull development,"
- "Use of isotretinoin during pregnancy may cause an under-development or over-development of the skull,"
- "Development of the ears may also be affected,"
- "The ears may not fully develop if isotretinoin is used during pregnancy. The outer ear may be deformed and the ear canal may be very small or absent entirely causing deformity,"
- "The eyes also may not develop fully,"
- "The eye socket may be very small or not develop at all causing facial deformity." (*Be Prepared. Be Protected*, 2013, p. 7–9)

In addition to the list of birth defects, women must sign a pledge acknowledging the risks. Accutane has serious risks, and the iPLEDGE program is set up so there is a standardized protocol to make all women aware of the risk of getting pregnant while having Accutane/isotretinoin in their systems. The iPLEDGE literature states:

> iPLEDGE Program is a set of steps all patients, doctors, and pharmacists must follow. The main goal is preventing pregnancy and birth defects, but both male patients and female patients must follow the iPLEDGE Program. The iPLEDGE Program is a single, shared Risk Evaluation and Mitigation Strategy (REMS) program for prescribing and dispensing all isotretinoin products (brand and generic products) and includes a pregnancy registry. To get isotretinoin, all patients must:

- Sign the Patient Information/Informed Consent form(s)
- Be able to keep appointments
- Agree to follow the iPLEDGE Program steps (*Be Prepared. Be Protected*, 2016, p. 3)

All the aforementioned information leads to several questions. Why is this level of warning and protocol with opioids and women of childbearing age not available? Why are women not warned about the potential dangers to their unborn children and about NAS?

In 2011, a national study on birth defects prevention suggested an association between maternal opioid-analgesic use and a number of congenital malformations, including neural tube defects such as spina bifida; heart issues such as conoventricular septal defects, hypoplastic left heart syndrome, and atrioventricular septal defects; and gastroschisis (Broussard et al., 2011, p. e311). In 2013, *Obstetrics and Gynecology* reported an increased risk of neural tube defects after first-trimester maternal opioid use (Yazdy et al., 2013, p. 838). These two studies, in addition to the ones mentioned earlier in this chapter, along with the well-established risk of neonatal withdrawal syndrome associated with opioid exposure in late pregnancy, bring to the forefront significant concerns about the use of opioids during pregnancy (Patrick et al., 2012, p. 1934).

Health communication messages are only useful if the message is reaching the affected population. Norwick and Morgan found only 43% of women were effectively counseled on proper birth-control methods while taking opioids (Holzman, 2018, p. 1). The National Institute on Drug Abuse reports, "every 25 minutes a baby is born suffering from opioid withdrawal" (U.S. Department of Health and Human Services & Centers for Disease Control and Prevention, 2015, p. 1). My goal is to issue a call to prescribers, doctors, women of childbearing age, and all health professionals to explain the risks opioids pose to women and their potential pregnancies.

Theory and praxis, working synergistically, may aid in spreading the message of the dangers that opioids present to neonates and women of childbearing age. The work of Coombs and Holladay was explored, specifically how their work contributes to a greater understanding of external perceptions of a crisis. Coombs and Holladay (2009) have studied how perception of a crisis is impacted by the inclusion of images when communicating about a crisis to the public. Coombs and Holladay concluded, "The inclusion of images featuring victims of a crisis could intensify attributions of crisis responsibility. As people consider the victims and sense greater danger, they could judge the organization as more responsible for the crisis" (Coombs and Holladay, 2009, p. 123). In summary, the inclusion of "real" people who have been impacted by the crisis does shape peoples' thoughts about the importance of holding those responsible for the crisis accountable. Coombs and Holladay's (2009) conclusion—that including images of actual victims increases the amount of responsibility people feel an organization has for "fixing" the problem—has been extracted from a myriad of formal case studies. If people could see images of a healthy baby in juxtaposition with a baby struggling to survive and plagued with NAS, prescribers and patients alike may think twice before taking or writing the prescription without strict adherence to birth-control methods.

Cian, Krishna, and Elder (2015) studied the impact of visual cues on behavior. Cian, Krishna, and Elder (2015) studied specifically how dynamic traffic signs can control driver behaviors. The authors concluded, "Our findings highlight the importance of incorporating dynamic elements into icon design to promote imagery and thereby elicit desired and responsible consumer behavior" (1426). The authors of the study note implications beyond driving, including using imagery to promote healthy behaviors and responsible consumer behaviors.

The campaigns to spread knowledge of the dangers of opioids must reach a wide audience because a baby is born with opioid addiction every 25 minutes in the United States, and 78 people die from opioid overdoses every day (U.S. Department of Health and Human Services, 2015, p. 1). Visual imagery may be one option to quickly alert women who were prescribed opioids of the potential dangers to a fetus.

6.5 HEALTH COMMUNICATION IMPLICATIONS

Prior to designing and implementing a health campaign similar to the one referenced in Section 6.4, consulting the health communication literature is important. The literature will assist in understanding the target population and effective methods to reach the at-risk population (Schiavo, 2013, p. 1–29; Viswanath, 2006, p. 216–219; Dutta-Bergman, 2005, p. 103–104). The health communication literature relates to the opioid crisis as it provides health care providers tools and suggestions on how to best discuss sensitive and personal information with patients, including risks and potential complications of taking medications.

Additionally, reviewing other successful health campaigns, such as the aforementioned example of Accutane, allows for a consideration of theory and praxis operating in an applied setting. The understanding of theory and praxis to construct a successful health campaign may aid in shifting the current paradigm of prescribing opioids for chronic pain to a new paradigm that views opioids as an inappropriate remedy for chronic pain (Chou, 2015; Lembke, 2016; Physicians for Responsible Opioid Prescription 2016).

Understanding who is the source of information and who is the receiver of the information allows for consideration of expertise and trustworthiness of the source (Kelley et al., 2016, p. 575). The communication framework developed by Goodnight (1982) allows for health information to be ascribed to three overarching spheres: technical, public, and personal (p. 218). The technical sphere includes those with a high-level knowledge or expertise: health professionals, authors in peer-reviewed journals, and scientific publications. The public sphere is made up of sources of information that are widely available: the Internet, mass media sources, and marketing and advertising. The personal sphere is based on relationships with family, friends, and colleagues. The spheres of knowledge can intersect—for example:

> websites directly convey research-based health information (public and technical) or when a trusted friend is also a physician (personal and technical) or when online forums act as social support (public and personal). The most trusted source is information received from the technical sphere, further highlighting

the need for improved doctor-patient communication dynamics. (Kelley et al., 2016, p. 575–580)

Considering the importance placed upon the technical sphere, beginning with doctor-patient communication is logical, as "communication is at the heart of who we are as human beings. It is our way of exchanging information; it also signifies our symbolic capability" (Rimal and Lapinski, 2009, p. 247). Effective interpersonal communication is important in a health care setting when communicating health care information (Schiavo, 2013, p. 102–103). Ineffective interpersonal communication between health care provider and patient can bring about "feelings of isolation and frustration," and in some instances "health information, or another kind of information, is misunderstood or blocked out because we cannot relate to the person who is speaking" (Schiavo, 2013, p. 103). The dynamics of interpersonal behavior must not be overlooked when communicating medical risk (Schiavo, 2013, p. 102–106).

Effective interpersonal communication in a treating relationship is important to patients' understanding the information presented to them and patients feeling comfortable asking the appropriate questions (Schiavo, 2013, p. 116–118). James Carey (1989) explains communication through the metaphor of transportation as a mode of moving information from one place to another (p. 15). This transmission metaphor is applicable from "imparting," "transporting," or "sending" information from one person or entity to another (p. 15). Carey (1989) explains that communication as a way of imparting information from one person to another in a mechanistic manner is limited, and he explains the nuance of communication through the metaphor of *ritual* (Carey, 1989, p. 18). Ritual is linked to an understanding of communication and to terms like *sharing, participation, association, fellowship, and the possession of a common faith* (Carey, 1989, p. 18). The metaphor of "ritual" allows for a representation of shared belief (Carey, 1989, p. 18). Carey's understanding of communication as a ritual informs health communication as the patient and health care provider work toward the goal of "commonness" of holistic health of body and mind. Carey's view of ritual communication can be applied so the patient and doctor move toward a common understanding of health at a time when opioids are being overprescribed. Application of Carey's ritual communication in a doctor-patient relationship would entail full disclosure of the risks of opioids, including a high risk of addiction and risks to future pregnancies for women. Additionally, maintaining a shared vision for what health is and how it is achieved is vital to the ongoing treating relationship.

Communication of health knowledge at the technical level can come from large institutions. The Centers for Disease Control and Prevention provides an informative document from every decade dating back to 1980, entitled *Healthy People*, that "provides science-based, national goals and objectives with 10-year targets designed to guide national health promotion and disease prevention efforts to improve the health of all people in the United States" (U.S. Department of Health and Human Services & Centers for Disease Control and Prevention, 2017). In 2010, for the first time, health communication was allocated a chapter in the "United States of America Healthy People 2010" objectives, denoting the importance of health communication (Rimal and Lapinski, 2009, p. 247). In "Healthy People 2010" in the U.S. public health agenda, "the scope of health communication in public health 'includes disease prevention, health promotion, health care policy, and the business of health care as well as enhancement of the quality of life and health of individuals within the community'" ("Healthy People" in Schiavo, 2013, p. 23–24). Health communication has the power to save lives, advance health outcomes, and increase the general health status of interested populations (p. 23).

There is a vast amount of information regarding personal health that is available through a myriad of channels. Viswanath states, "Combined with revolutionary developments in the biomedical sciences and telecommunications, plenty of health information and delivery channels now exist" (p. 216). A review of the health communication literature allows for insight into the effectiveness of health campaigns and the impact the health campaigns can have on an intended audience.

Two main challenges are articulated in the literature in the construction and reception of a health campaign. The first challenge is the need to translate scientific information to a usable format by translating scientific jargon into language that can be easily understood by the intended audience (Viswanath, 2016, p. 217; Dutta-Bergman, 2005, p. 103–104). The second challenge is making the information available to those who need it, "regardless of their social class, cultural, geographic, and individual backgrounds" (Viswanath, 2016, p. 218; Dutta-Bergman, 2005, p.103–104). Dutta-Bergman (2005) explains the vast dichotomy of the "haves and the have nots" through a metaphor of a "societal chasm" (p. 104). Several scholars have articulated that socioeconomic status and education level impact the reception of health information (Viswanath, 2006; Schiavo, 2013; Dutta-Bergman, 2005).

Viswanath (2006) explains, "Profound disparities in disease burden among different social classes, possibly partly attributed to lack of information. For example, even as the overall burden of cancer is steadily falling, the decline varies for groups of different racial/ethnic and socioeconomic backgrounds" (Kawachi and Kroenke quoted in Viswanath, 2006, p. 219; Krieger, Lynch, and Kaplan quoted in Viswanath, 2006, p. 219). Not having access to health information and not having the financial means to make said changes can be deadly as "higher cancer incidences in minorities and lower socioeconomic groups also tend to have high rates of death due to cancer" (Viswanath, 2006, p. 219). Understanding the vast discrepancies in health literacy between the "haves" and the "have nots" allows health communication professionals and medical professionals to collaborate on the best practice to reach the intended audience.

Viswanath (2006), Schiavo (2013), and Dutta-Bergman (2005) have articulated how socioeconomic status and education level impact health literacy, and this is relevant to the opioid crisis. The highest levels of NAS in the United States are also in the poorest and most rural states like Kentucky, West Virginia, Alabama, and Mississippi (White, 2016). Rural parts of Kentucky have experienced an exceptionally high number of NAS cases, and "within Kentucky, rates in Appalachia are 50 per 1,000, or more than twice that of the state's overall rate" (Brown in White, 2016, p. 1).

Dr. Joshua Brown, a researcher at the University of Kentucky College of Pharmacy who studies NAS, reports, "Although the population is lower in rural areas, the number of NAS births is equal to that of the metro areas simply because the rate is so high" (White, 2016, p. 1). Brown believes lack of money and education has contributed to this issue: "We expect the rural aspect is really driving it as well as the socioeconomic factors associated with that" (Brown in White, 2016, p. 1). The lack of money, the lack of education, and the lack of health literacy are contributing to the occurrence of NAS in the United States, especially in places like Kentucky, West Virginia, Alabama, and Mississippi. A health campaign informed by theory and praxis would be sensitive to the needs of the most at-risk population, and in this case, it is the rural and impoverished.

6.6 HEALTH THEORIES THAT MAY OFFER INSIGHT INTO THE OPIOID CRISIS

Diffusion of Innovation Theory

Several theories inform health communication and can be used when considering curtailing the opioid crisis. Diffusion of Innovation Theory, initially developed by Everett Rogers in the 1960s, classifies people into subgroups based on their willingness and propensity to accept and adopt innovation: innovators, early adopters, early majority, late majority, and laggards (Rogers, 1983). Rogers provides an example of a village in Peru where the drinking water was causing disease, and the cure was boiling the water prior to use. Rogers reported only eleven women followed the orders and boiled the water, and he explains different characteristics associated with those people who made the changes first and with those who resisted the advice to boil the water. Roger's theory does not presuppose the information trickles down from the top to the bottom; rather, communication of information is "a process in which participants create and share information with one another in order to reach a mutual understanding" (Waisbord, 2001, p. 5).

Roger's theory considers that change is a gradual process of diffusion: "Diffusion is the process by which an innovation is communicated through certain channels over time among the members of a social system. It is a special type of communication, in that the messages are concerned with new ideas" (Rogers, 1983, p. 5).

The diffusion of Innovation Theory is particularly relevant when studying the opioid crisis because the innovators and the early adopters, such as Dr. Lembke, realized opioids flowing from doctors to patients were of serious concern. Early adopters who were seeing patients becoming addicted to opioids in droves sounded the alarm to other doctors and encouraged responsible prescribing. The early adopters were in the minority in the 1990s. Lembke writes, "By the late 1990s, I realized I had one of two choices: I could continue to ignore my patients' substance use problems, or I could figure out how to target and treat addiction" (2016, p. 2). During the late 1990s, the paradigm most other doctors were ascribing to was that opioids were indeed the cure for chronic pain. Lembke (2016) understood the risks of opioids; she was an early adopter and changed her clinical praxis. Lembke began to treat opioid addiction before the issue was widely published; furthermore, she wrote a book detailing her experiences and explaining the medical literature as support (2016, p. 1–45). Lembke (2016) allowed her ideas to be diffused to others through peer-reviewed literature and books, slowly reaching those who were reluctant to change.

The Diffusion of Innovation Theory describes five primary characteristics of the innovation: relative advantage, compatibility, complexity, trialability, and observability (Rogers, 1983). Wagner et al. (2020) take these characteristics and explain them in medical terms. Relative advantage represents the degree to which the innovation is perceived as better than the current standard of care. Compatibility represents the degree to which the innovation is compatible with values, experiences, and needs of the clinical adopters. Complexity represents how difficult the innovation is to implement. Trialability has to do with the degree to which the innovation can be tried and subsequently modified, while observability represents the degree to which the adoption of the innovation can be seen by others.

There have been several studies completed about administering take-home Narcan to people who are addicted to opioids through the lens of the Diffusion of Innovation Theory (Wagner et al., 2020; Bowles and Lankenau, 2019). Wagner et al. (2020) concluded complexity was an issue, "Our findings suggest that educational and academic detailing efforts are required and should focus on increasing the confidence among ER staff that THN (take-home Narcan) and the information provided by MROTs (mobile recovery outreach teams) can be an effective and lifesaving intervention for opioid overdose patients" (p. 102). Bowles and Lankenau (2018) also found complexity to be an issue, "The present study qualitatively examined the diffusion process of OOPP [opioid overdose prevention programs] among 30 persons who inject drugs (PWIDs) in an opioid-saturated community. Purposive sampling was used to recruit participants into three groups based on familiarity with the OOPP. Findings revealed that participants often adopted the OOPP, which was offered by a local harm-reduction organization, if first exposed by staff hosting and implementing it" (p. 345).

Health Belief Theory

Another theory from the health communication literature that has implications to the opioid crisis is the health belief model. It involves understanding health risks and vulnerability to the risk. According to Schiavo (2013), "the major assumption of this model is that in order to engage in healthy behaviors, key groups need to be aware of their risk for severe or life-threatening diseases and perceive that the benefits of behavior change outweigh potential barriers or other negative aspects of recommended actions" (p. 40). The health belief model was developed in the early 1950s by the U.S. Public Health Service in an attempt to understand why people were not partaking in preventative screenings for asymptomatic disease and why people failed to comply with prescribed medical treatment plans (Janz and Becker, 1984, p. 2). Janz and Becker (1984) wrote a monograph—*The Health Belief Model and Personal Health Behavior*—that summarized research findings of why individuals did or did not engage in health-related behaviors (1). The health belief model is based upon perception and education of the risks of a certain health behavior.

Schiavo (2013) describes the following key parts of the health belief model:

- Perceived susceptibility: The individual's perception of whether he or she is at risk for contracting a specific illness or health problem
- Perceived severity: The subjective feeling on whether the specific illness or health problem can be severe (for example, permanently impair physical or mental functions) or is life-threatening and therefore worthy of one's attention
- Perceived benefits: The individual's perceptions of the advantages of adopting recommended actions that would eventually reduce the risk for disease severity, morbidity, and mortality
- Perceived barriers: The individual's perceptions of the costs of and obstacles to adopting recommended actions (includes economic costs as well as other kinds of lifestyle sacrifices)

- Cues to action: Public or social events that can signal the importance of taking action (for example, a neighbor who is diagnosed with the same disease, or a mass media campaign)
- Self-efficacy: The individual's confidence in his or her ability to perform and sustain the recommended behavior with little or no help from others (Schiavo, 2013, p. 40–41).

The health belief model is often referred to as a risk-learning model (Pechmann, 2001, p. 189). Pechmann (2001) elaborates that the health belief model is a "risk learning model because the goal is to teach new information about health risks and the behaviors that minimize those risks" (p. 189). The health belief model emphasizes the role of learning as necessary though not always sufficient for change (Schiavo, 2013, p. 41). The health belief model is important to the opioid crisis because many clinicians believed the risk of becoming addicted to opioids was low (Porter and Jick in Moghe, 2016).

The health belief model is particularly relevant in dispelling the myth to patients and doctors that opioids are not addictive, as opioids are highly addictive and not appropriate as a treatment for chronic pain (Chou, 2015). Jane Porter and Dr. Hershel Jick concluded after performing an analysis of approximately 11,000 people that "the development of addiction is rare in medical patients with no history of addiction" (Porter and Jick in Moghe, 2016). About six years later in May of 1986, Portenoy and Foley published a study in the journal *Pain* where they conclude "that opioid maintenance therapy can be a safe, salutary, and more humane alternative to the options of surgery or no treatment in those patients with intractable non-malignant pain and no history of drug abuse" (p. 171). The low risk of addiction to opioids has been disproven, as 78 people die every day from an opioid overdose due to severe opioid addiction (Enomoto in Murthy III).

Theory of Reasoned Action

The Theory of Reasoned Action is attributed to Ajzen and Fishbein. The theory of reasoned action approach that Martin Fishbein pioneered has emerged as one of the dominant conceptual frameworks for predicting, explaining, and changing human social behavior (Ajzen, 2012, p. 11). Two major factors contribute to changing behaviors. The first factor is attitude. A person's attitude can be defined as positive or negative toward a behavior, concept, or idea (Ajzen, 2012). The second factor is subjective norms about behavior. A subjective norm is defined as an opinion that loved ones, friends, family, or colleagues have about a potential behavior (Ajzen, 2012). A subjective norm is influenced by whether a person may believe significant others will approve of his or her potential action (Schiavo, 2013, p. 44). The theory of reasoned action is useful in analyzing and identifying reasons for action and what may change people's attitudes toward a health behavior (Schiavo, 2013, p. 45).

6.7 CONCLUSIONS AND CONNECTIONS

One of the main goals of this project was to explore the connection between the historical moment and the opioid crisis. Modernity's commitment to the grand narrative of science creates challenges, opportunities, and a false sense of hope that science and logic can solve most problems (Arnett, 2012, p. i–iii). The hope that pharmacology can relieve all pain is a myth (Morris, 1991). David Morris is a writer and scholar and an emeritus professor of literature at the University of Virginia. Morris is well respected by the medical community as he was asked to speak at conferences, including the American Academy of Pain Management. David Morris explains that illness is "situated at the crossroads of biology and culture" (p. 71). Morris further explains illness is tied to the historical moment, and how one "cures illness" is also tied to the historical moment. In turn, the historical moment is tied to culture (Morris, 1991). In this particular historical moment, people have become conditioned to reach for pills to cure pain. Culture is what pulls people "irresistibly toward the medicine cabinet, as if pills and tablets held a kind of magnetic, eternal attraction for the unseen torments of a bad back or any other type of pain" (Morris, 1991, p. 2). Morris (1991) further articulates the impossibility of separating mental and physical pain in the "Myth of Two Pains" (p. 9). Morris, Gadamer, and Lembke all acknowledge the connection between mind and body, as well as the need to understand "pain" as an experience and not merely as a nerve sensation.

Another connection to the historical moment is the large amount of power institutions have in modernity. The American Pain Society, the Joint Commission, and the Veterans Administration convey power and prestige (Lembke, 2016). All three of these organizations recognized pain as a vital sign, prompting swift interventions including prescribing of opioids and numeric rating scales for measurements of pain (Lembke, 2016). Foucault's (1982) body of work, especially *The Subject and Power,* explores the construct of power and how power impacts society. Foucault (1982) explores the medical profession's power and writes the medical profession is criticized "for an uncontrolled power over people's bodies, their health and their life and death" (p. 780). Power structures in the doctor-patient relationship are relevant in the way many patients trusted their doctors to be objective and to prescribe medications solely for the purpose of healing.

Social practices are used to reinforce knowledge, and discourse constructs the topic (Hall, 2001, p. 72) The social practice of a patient entering a doctor's office and leaving with opioid prescriptions constructs the idea that chronic pain is cured by opioids. The opioid companies successfully created "pseudoknowledge " linking opioids as a cure for chronic pain and continually reinforced the practice of treating chronic pain with pills in all types of advertising. Advertising becomes a source of episteme constructed by the institutions belonging to the pharmaceutical industry.

Foucault (1980) writes:

> I would define the episteme retrospectively as the strategic apparatus which permits separating out from among all the statements which are possible those that will be acceptable within, I won't say a scientific theory, but a field of scientificity, and which it is possible to say are true or false. The episteme is the "apparatus" which makes possible the separation, not of the true from the false, but of what may from what may not be characterized as scientific. (p. 197)

Big Pharma and Pain Societies were a part of the institutional power-diffusing "episteme."

Doctors clearly abused their power and betrayed the "ethic" of the profession. Fritz argues, "Ethical norms provide a basis for self-evaluation of professions as communities of practice, defining the 'good' that is protected and promoted by a given profession" (Fritz, 2013, p. 5). The "good" of the medical profession is healing, and that ethic is violated when physicians prescribe opioids for profit (Brookbank, 2017; U.S. Attorney's Office, 2017). Ethical norms were violated as pain societies, who represented themselves as objective, were funded by the pharmaceutical industry. Lembke (2016) reports that "the American Pain Foundation, a medical society for doctors who treat pain, received 90 percent of its $5 million funding in 2010 from the drug and medical device industry" (p. 62). Arguably, the pain societies betrayed their own members.

The other goal of this project is to explore implications of the opioid crisis to communication and rhetorical studies. The rhetorical nature of science and the explanation of how bias, language, and persuasion shift paradigms are relevant to understanding how the opioid crisis began (Kuhn, 1970). In the early 1970s and 1980s, nurses and doctors were trained to prescribe minimal opioids (Meldrum, 2016, p. 1365). Purdue Pharma and their paid "thought leaders" influenced unsuspecting doctors who were attending medical conferences in the hopes of getting objective information to include into their praxis; rather, the doctors at the medical conferences received pro-opioid rhetoric in the hopes of boosting sales. These trained speakers or "thought leaders" gave lectures about the "appropriate use of opioids, including oxycodone, the active ingredient in OxyContin, to their colleagues in various settings, such as local medical conferences and grand round presentations in hospitals involving physicians, residents, and interns" (U.S. General Accounting Office, 2003, p. 22). Unfortunately, the risks of addiction were not adequately covered in the presentations, and doctors began liberally prescribing.

Framing techniques such as relying upon metaphors, catch phrases, and narratives, as explained by Fairhurst and Sarr, create frames of interpretation with the hope of shaping one's views. Framing techniques also shifted the paradigm from minimal opioid prescribing to liberal prescribing of opioids (U.S. General Accounting Office, 2003). Creating the construct of "opiophobia" framed doctors who refused to prescribe opioids as insensitive to their patients' pain (Lembke, 2016, p. 63). This project brings to the forefront ethical implications, specifically privileging profits ahead of people, with regard to Purdue Pharma. The lack of regard for people and Purdue Pharma's refusal in explaining the "real" risk of addiction and opioids suggest a starting point for a future project.

Another starting point for future implications of this project may be the insurance industry's lack of willingness to cover the best-known alternative to opioids, intensive programming with therapeutic options. This project highlighted the Kaiser program in California, which frames chronic pain as a construct with physical, emotional, and behavioral elements. The program services include pain education classes, family sessions, aftercare program with exercise, medication management, acupuncture, and biofeedback. Meldrum (2018) points out:

> The best-known alternative to opioids is a multidisciplinary team approach involving reliance on physical and psychological therapies, including cognitive-behavioral therapy, relaxation and pain coping skills training, and self-hypnosis. While such methods can be highly successful, many third-party payers regard them as too costly; insurance coverage is usually inadequate, and only major medical centers can support such programs. Fewer than 200,000 patients currently participate in multidisciplinary treatment. (p. 1365)

A multidisciplinary approach may be expensive and time consuming, but that may be the only mechanism to address the Myth of Two Pains and to realize emotional pain can manifest in physical ways (Morris, 1991).

The implications of the opioid crisis are now reaching the family unit and children. The health and well-being of the individual has implications for the family, and the health of the family has implications for the community as a whole. Families are being torn apart; parents are tending to their addictions, neglecting their children; and foster care systems are becoming overwhelmed (Collier, 2018, p. 18). The family unit has implications for health of the individual family members, and as the health of the family unit suffers, so can the health of the members of the family (House et al. in Albrecht and Goldsmith

2003, p. 326). Future generations are now being affected by their parents' opioid usage; one must stop and realize opioids are not the solution. Perhaps one of the most important implications from this project is to suggest all women, regardless of socioeconomic status and level of health literacy, be warned of the dangers opioids pose to her and any future children. When taking opioids during pregnancy, NAS is not the only concern; the larger concern is the complete dysfunction that opioid addiction brings and the personal chaos it creates for addicts and their families.

Chapter Seven

An Ecological Perspective of the Medicolegal Ramifications and Corporate Reactions to the Opioid Crisis

Ecology is the study of the interaction between organisms and their environments. The opioid crisis presents a rare opportunity to study the unique ecological system that propagated the opioid crisis, and the relationship of influence between doctors, patients, and opioid manufacturers. Street (2003) explored the ecological relationships in a medical context focusing on the interactions between doctor and patient. Discourse between a physician and patient is sacred and has been studied and protected since antiquity with the advent of the Hippocratic Oath in the fifth century. This discourse is relevant when examining the opioid crisis. Street (2003) explains "the primary activity is talk as the provider and patient exchange information about health-related concerns; make decisions about medical care; and, in the best of cases, establish or maintain a relationship characterized by rapport, trust, and respect" (p. 66). Interpersonal communication has been the primary lens applied to studying the discourse between the doctor and patient (Street, 2003). Pain societies, physicians, pharmaceutical companies, marketing agencies working to promote opioids, activists working against the prescribing of opioids, the federal government, and patients are all important parts of the crisis and have influenced conversations between patient and doctor. This chapter looks at the role of the interpersonal relationship, the organization, and overview of trends surrounding the corporate reaction to the opioid crisis.

As a result of the opioid crisis, the trusting rapport between patient and doctor may have been contaminated by an outside force. These conversations may have been influenced in an insidious manner by opioid manufacturers and their aggressive marketing. This chapter considers the rhetoric of opioid manufacturers influencing the conversations and interactions between doctor and patient. Street (2003) proposes an ecological model of communication in medical encounters. The ecological model begins with the interpersonal communication and broadens out to make room for considerations such as the media context, the cultural context, the political-legal context, and the organizational context. When accounting for outside societal forces, the analysis of the doctor-patient discourse becomes perhaps easier to contextualize within a broader rhetorical landscape. Moreover, this chapter seeks to explore the ongoing litigation in the attempt to bring forth accountability and liability on behalf of the patients who became addicted.

7.1 INFLUENTIAL RHETORICAL VARIABLES IN DOCTOR-PATIENT RELATIONSHIPS

Trust in a clinical setting is a vital part of the doctor-patient relationship. Roter and Hall (2004) conceptualize the dynamic between doctor and patient as a partnership; they write "partnership-building occurs when the physician actively facilitates patient participation in the medical visit and/or attempts to equalize status by assuming a less dominating stance within the relationship" (p. 505). Hall, Horgan, Stein, and Roter (2002) studied the interactions between patients and doctors and found the more the patient liked the doctor the more willing they were to follow their advice, and patients who liked their doctors reported higher levels of feeling healthy in the form of self-reporting their perception of their overall health. Roter and Hall (2004) explain the dynamic between patient and doctor can be influenced by gender, as "the patients of female physicians spoke more overall, disclosed more biomedical and psychosocial information, and made more positive statements to their physicians than did the patients of male physicians" (p. 497).

Likability and gender were not the only influences at work when doctors and patients discussed opioids. Apparently "doctors didn't question what they were told by pharmaceutical representatives and on continuing medical-education courses about prescription opioids, in part because of a lack of experience," says Stephen Bernard, a palliative-care specialist at the University of North Carolina at Chapel Hill. "Physicians don't get a lot of good training in pain management," he says (Bernard in DeWeerdt, 2019, para 9). The opioid manufacturers and pain societies funded by the opioid manufacturers capitalized on this and pushed opioids to physicians as the best choice for chronic pain, when in fact the medical evidence does not support this. For example, in 2003 the *New England Journal of Medicine* published a review article on prescribing opioids for chronic pain and the authors of the article were misled by the very pain societies that were funded by the opioid manufacturers, stating "Key organizations that strongly support the use of opioids to treat chronic pain have published consensus statements to guide physicians in prescribing these drugs" (p. 1944). Additionally, in 2003, the *New England Journal of Medicine* did mention that some doctors had concerns about the use and the marginal benefits of opioids for chronic pain, and minimal effect on function, but the journal noted this was a minority view (p. 1944). The rhetorical position of the broader medical literature in the early 2000s was in large part pro-opioid, and many of the doctors who published these articles were "thought leaders" (paid speakers by the opioid manufacturers who spoke only about the positives of opioids) or doctors who attended the conferences sponsored by opioid manufacturers (Lembke, 2016). Opioid manufacturers sponsored continuing education seminars, provided trips for doctors to desirable locations, and aggressively set up sales representatives to visit doctors' offices; sales reps often left gifts and designed commercials to play in waiting rooms.

In 2016—a bit more than a decade later—another article was published in the *New England Journal of Medicine* which shifted the rhetoric; it warned that opioids may not be the best treatment for chronic pain. The *New England Journal of Medicine* reported, "However, two major facts can no longer be questioned. First, opioid analgesics are widely diverted and improperly used, and the widespread use of the drugs has resulted in a national epidemic of opioid overdose deaths and addictions. More than a third (37%) of the 44,000 drug-overdose deaths that were reported in 2013 (the most recent year for which estimates are available) were attributable to pharmaceutical opioids; heroin accounted for an additional 19%. At the same time, there has been a parallel increase in the rate of opioid addiction, affecting approximately 2.5 million adults in 2014. Second, the major source of diverted opioids is physician prescriptions. For these reasons, physicians and medical associations have begun questioning prescribing practices for opioids, particularly as they relate to the management of chronic pain" (Volkow & McLellan, 2016, p. 1253). In 2016, in JAMA, an article appeared reviewing the CDC guidelines and that recommendations from the CDC were clear, "Of primary importance, nonopioid therapy is preferred for treatment of chronic pain" (Dowell et al., 2016, p. 1624). The shifting rhetoric about the benefits of opioids for chronic pain in the past decade is worthy of scholarly investigation. The next section seeks to explore why the rhetoric was pro-opioid for chronic pain and how society is attempting to hold those with power and influence accountable through legal channels.

7.2 LAWSUITS

The opioid crisis has claimed many lives and has wreaked havoc on many families. People are angry, need help, and have turned to the legal system to seek justice. Beckman, Markakis, Suchman, and Frankel (1994) found that the individual decision to sue in a medical setting was heavily associated with a perceived lack of caring by physicians and a lack of collaboration in health care delivery. However, the lawsuits revolving around the opioid crisis are in large part brought on by states, communities, and major medical centers against pharmaceutical companies. The individual suing the doctor is a small minority of the lawsuits. According to the CDC, more than 67,000 people died from drug overdoses in 2018, making it a leading cause of injury-related death in the United States. Of those deaths, almost 70% involved a prescription or illicit opioid (CDC, 2020). Many states are in the process or have sued opioid drug manufacturers.

Opioid manufacturers were first sued in early 2000s by West Virginia, Kentucky, and the federal government. "In 2007, Purdue executives pleaded guilty in the federal case to falsely advertising OxyContin as 'less addictive' and 'less subject to abuse and diversion' than other pain medications. The company agreed to pay $600 million in criminal and civil fines to the federal government, and $20 million to 26 states and the District of Columbia" (Vestal, 2019, para 8). This did not deter the opioid manufacturers as opioid overprescribing and opioid misuse disorder continued to spiral out of control.

In March 2017, Oklahoma Attorney General Mike Hunter and Attorney Michael Burrage announced a major lawsuit against more than a dozen pharmaceutical companies that manufacture and distribute opioid pain pills (Savage, 2017). Attorney General Hunter has strongly come out against opioids and the drug companies who have marketed them as safe. It took approximately two years for Oklahoma to get money from Purdue, but the company did pay. "Purdue appears to have concluded that it was less risky to settle the Oklahoma case than have the allegations publicly aired against it during a televised trial and face exposure to what could have been an astronomical jury verdict," said Abbe R. Gluck, a professor at Yale Law School who directs the Solomon Center for Health Policy and Law" (Hoffman, 2019, para 3). "OxyContin maker Purdue Pharma LP and members of the wealthy Sackler family that own the company reached a $270 million settlement to resolve a lawsuit brought by the state of Oklahoma accusing the drug maker of fueling an opioid abuse epidemic" and this money is going to help people struggling with opioid addiction (Raymond, 2019). The deceptive marketing practices were highlighted in the complaint against Purdue. The

$270 million settlement covers Purdue, which left claims against Johnson & Johnson and Teva Pharmaceutical open (Raymond, 2019).

It was not until three months later in June of 2019, that a judge approved a revised $85 million settlement between Teva Pharmaceuticals and Oklahoma, which the state said it would use in its battle agains the opioid epidemic. Teva agreed to not hire or employ in any manner salespeople to endorse opioids in the state and Teva promised to refrain from using lectures or speakers to promote opioids (Drash, 2019).

A few months later, Judge Thad Balkman of Oklahoma, on Monday, August 26, 2019, ruled that "Johnson & Johnson had intentionally played down the dangers and oversold the benefits of opioids and ordered it to pay the state $572 million in the first trial of a drug manufacturer for the destruction wrought by prescription painkillers" (Hoffman, 2019, para 1).

On December 17, 2019, Michigan was the first state to sue major opioid distributors as drug dealers. Michigan first filed a lawsuit against Cardinal Health Inc., McKesson Corporation, AmerisourceBergen Drug Corporation, and Walgreens in Wayne County Circuit Court (Rossman-McKinney, 2019). Michigan Attorney General Dana Nessel said, "These companies knowingly and deliberately used their licenses to distribute drugs in our state without controls," Nessel further explained, "This was not only negligent; it was unlawful, a public nuisance and, as a result, their actions subject these companies to liability under Michigan's Drug Dealer Liability Act" (Rossman-McKinney, 2019).

Other states are following suit: "We are suing the giant, the pharma lord who created OxyContin," Pennsylvania Attorney General Josh Shapiro said at a news conference on May 14, 2019 (Winter and Schapiro, 2019, para 3). Johnson & Johnson, Purdue Pharma, Teva Pharmaceutical, and other companies promoted their opioid products aggressively (DeWeerdt, 2019, para 9). "They lobbied lawmakers, sponsored continuing medical-education courses, funded professional and patient organizations and sent representatives to visit individual doctors. During all of these activities, they emphasized the safety, efficacy and low potential for addiction of prescription opioids" (DeWeerdt, 2019, para 9).

It appears the litigation has grown so large that a class action lawsuit has been formed. The National Prescription Opiate Litigation also known as the MDL No. 2804 (Northern District, Ohio), is a group litigation which includes more than 2,000 cases. This is the first time this type of litigation has been used under Federal Rule of Civil Procedure 23. The rationale for this form of suit is combining "all cities and counties together as a Negotiation Class gives them maximum negotiating power, makes the negotiation of comprehensive settlements a more practical process, enables Defendants to know the group with which they are negotiating, and enables Class Members to vote on resulting settlement offers" (In Re: National Prescription Opiate Litigation, 2020, para 3). This litigation combines a myriad of communities from all over the United States.

Judge Polster of the U.S. District Court of Northern District of Ohio. Eastern Division was assigned as transferee judge, and he is overseeing the litigation. From Judge Polster's opinion and order filed September 26, 2019, it appears the plaintiffs are "governmental entities—Cities and Counties from across the country, as well as Indian Tribes." Judge Polster adds that other plaintiffs include "hospitals, third-party payors, putative classes of individuals, and others" (Polster, 2019, p. 1). Polster notes this litigation is the "most complex and important group of cases ever" because of both the "magnitude" and "significance" of the opioid crisis (Polster, 2019, p. 1). Judge Polster has encouraged the parties to reach a settlement and not litigate. A negotiation class means any settlement must be approved by 75% of the class. As of July 2020, the litigation is ongoing, and a global settlement has not been reached.

There are locations that have opted out of the negotiation class, especially those areas that have been particularly hard hit by the crisis. Reuter's reports, "However, the 541 local governments that opted out included Florida's Palm Beach County and counties in West Virginia, according to attorneys, raising the prospect that companies could face expensive trials even if they settled with the class" (Hals, 2019, para 3). Suing the pharmaceutical companies will not bring back those who have died from an overdose, but many feel that the companies should pay to *clean up* the mess they have left behind and help offset the costs of drug rehab.

7.3 THE FAMILY BEHIND PURDUE

At the time of the opioid crisis peak, the Sackler family was one of the richest families in the United States, and the family owns 100% of Purdue Pharma. The Sackler family came under a lot of public scrutiny for their role in the opioid crisis since "oxycodone has been a major factor—perhaps *the* major factor—in the rise of the opioid epidemic" (Van Way, 2019, para 3). OxyContin is manufactured by Purdue Pharma; it is a trade name for a long-acting form of oxycodone.

In 2015, the Sackler family was ranked by *Forbes Magazine* as having approximately $14 billion, and the Sackler family net worth was greater than the Busches, Mellons, and Rockefellers (Morrell, 2016). The Sackler family was not always that wealthy. The Sackler brothers, Arthur born in 1913, Mortimer born in 1916, and Raymond born in 1920, were born to immigrant grocers in Brooklyn, New York. Each brother attended medical school and all three brothers became psychiatrists. Arthur Sackler was known for his marketing genius as he was one of the first doctors who worked to invent complex advertising campaigns to push pharmaceuticals direct to doctors. As the Medical Advertising Hall of Fame declared in 1998, "No single individual did more to shape the character of medical advertising than the multitalented Dr. Arthur Sackler. His seminal contribution was bringing the full power of advertising and promotion to pharmaceutical marketing" (Podolsky et al., 2019, p. 25). Arthur Sackler directed Pfizer's marketing campaigns for the powerful antibiotics Terramycin and Tetracyn, commonly referred to as tetracycline. Arthur Sackler's aggressive sales plans included growth of the drug sales force, as the sales force grew from eight salespeople in 1950 to 2,000 sales people by 1957. "Doctors in nearly every specialty were persuaded to consider conditions ranging from upper respiratory infections to urinary tract infections as necessitating antibiotics" (Podolsky et al., 2019, para 4). Sackler's sales force was successful and led to strong profits for Pfizer; some would argue the aggressive sales force led to the overprescribing of strong antibiotics.

In 1952, life changed for the Sackler brothers, and they bought Purdue-Frederick, a small New York City drug company, which later grew to become Purdue Pharma (Sales, 2019). In the 1950s the company mainly produced laxatives, but that changed with the advent of a marketing scheme to push the benefits of a controlled-release opioid, OxyContin, in the 1990s. Investigators cite, "because the dangers of addiction to OxyContin were downplayed or kept hidden—the Sackler name has become synonymous with controversy" (Sales, 2019). The Food and Drug Administration had allowed Purdue Pharma to make a unique claim for OxyContin—"that, as a long-acting opioid, it might be less likely to cause abuse and addiction than shorter-acting painkillers like Percocet" (Meier, 2018a, para 3). OxyContin's time-release design ("contin" was short for "continuous") gave it an advantage over older painkillers (i.e., Percocet). "But Purdue Pharma also claimed that OxyContin would be less appealing than traditional painkillers to drug abusers" (Meier, 2018a, p. 9).

Purdue Pharma focused on this point and in 1996 it launched an enormous marketing campaign for OxyContin based on that claim. The aggressive marketing tactics included offering doctors all-expenses-paid trips to pain-management seminars. Purdue formed its own speaker bureau with clinicians propagandizing about the positives of the drug, advertised in medical journals, sponsored online sites for chronic pain, gave away a wide variety of branded merchandise, and Purdue produced and distributed promotional videos with satisfied patients discussing their satisfaction with OxyContin. The Purdue videos were distributed to doctors across the country to play in their waiting rooms. Moreover, the "The marketing of OxyContin relied on an empirical circularity: the company convinced doctors of the drug's safety with literature that had been produced by doctors who were paid, or funded, by the company" (Keefe, 2017, para 24).

Quickly, people were crushing the pills that alleged to be "slow-releasing" and when doing so a huge dose of opioids was released in the system creating a path for drug abuse and addiction. Meier (2018a) explains that the top executives at Purdue knew this was occurring and did not do anything to stop it. Meier (2018a) reported, "In 2007, the Purdue Pharma executives had pleaded guilty to misdemeanor charges that held them liable solely as the company's 'responsible' corporate officers and did not accuse them of any personal wrongdoing" (para 11). The Sackler family amassed an enormous fortune from the sales of OxyContin, and it is not surprising marketing efforts were paramount in their financial *success*. The insidious nature of the actions of the Sacklers who controlled Purdue infiltrated "the prescribing practices and of the approach to pain recommended in clinical journals, medical curricula, and professional guidelines" (Podolsky, Herzberg, and Greene et al., 2019, para 1). The Sackler family in 2018 had eight family members on the board but in 2019 there were no family members left on the board (Sales, 2019). The Sackler family was once known for its philanthropic efforts as the family name appears on many museums and universities throughout the world. However, many prestigious institutions are now refusing gifts from the family, citing the organization does not want to be connected to a family at the center of the opioid crisis.

Even with the expansive lawsuits pending against Purdue Pharma and the Sackler family it appears the family's wealth will be left intact. The bankruptcy court has expansive powers, and it may benefit the Sackler family. The *New York Times* reported, "The Sacklers would walk away with an estimated several billion of OxyContin profits while leaving unresolved a crucial question asked by victims and their families" (Posner and Brubaker, 2020, para 5). The legal precedent appears to be on the Sackler's side. In a 1985 case in which the A. H. Robins Company, the manufacturer of the Dalkon Shield contraceptive device, filed for bankruptcy and the court extended legal protections to the owners of the company and their family members, even after lawyers alleged the family hid dangers of the product (Posner and Brubaker, 2020, para 5). Because of the case log largely being on the side of the Sackler family, many legal scholars predict the Sackler family fortune will be largely protected from the lawsuits.

On November 17, 2020, bankruptcy Judge Drain approved the controversial settlement leaving the majority of the Sackler's wealth intact and focusing most of the penalties on the Purdue corporation. "Under terms approved by Judge Robert Drain, Purdue Pharma will plead guilty to three felony counts of criminal wrongdoing" (Mann, 2020, para 1). The Purdue corporate structure will most likely be reorganized so that profits from all opioid sales fund programs aimed at alleviating the addiction crisis. The focus of the penalties is on the corporation and not people, though the Sackler family will forfeit $225 million of their own money as part of the litigation, which is a small fraction of their remarkable wealth (Mann, 2020). There is tremendous public outcry regarding the terms of the settlement.

7.4 VOICES OF DISSENT

Public protests historically have had a critical role in the enactment of democracy and a public act of the expression of the will of the people (Cottle, 2008). Tulke (2020) explains the important connections between social movements and the visual arts. She writes, "creative interventions into public space have the potential to stage meaningful encounters between city dwellers and the urban landscape they inhabit, inscribing alternative histories and possibilities into the very surface of the city" (p. 122). Dissent is part of a healthy democracy and is the balancing point between "stability and change" (Ivie, 2015, p. 46). Ivie (2015) notes that true democracy cannot exist if public opinion is shaped only from ruling elites. Ivie (2015) continues and explains the value of dissent, "The constitutive value of dissent itself, as an ongoing exercise in democratic engagement, is less frequently recognized and insufficiently understood for the demand it makes on rhetorical invention" (p. 47). Dissent encourages democratic engagement and dissent requires discourse. The dissenters must air their grievances and communicate ideas that they perceive will remedy the situations. Dissent is a rhetorical act of invention (Ivie, 2015). The public acts of dissent against the Sackler family, Purdue Pharma, and the legal settlement include the visual arts, and creative interventions in public spaces. Exploring these acts of dissent help us to understand the concerns of those who feel wronged.

Nan Goldin, an activist in New York City, organized a group called Sackler Pain (P.A.I.N.), and this organization focuses on getting the word out that the Sackler family is not being held accountable. Nan Goldin created public awareness of the Purdue Pharma's role in opioid crisis by staging a creative *die-in* in the Sackler Wing of the Metropolitan Museum of Art. On March 18, 2018, Goldfin organized a myriad of people to gather around ponds at the Temple of Dendur and instead of tossing coins into the water people tossed empty prescription pill containers (Russeth, 2019). The people then dropped to the ground chanting "Sacklers lie. People die" (Russeth, 2019, para 10). Goldin has staged other dramatic live artistic protests at other prestigious museums, including the Guggenheim in New York City. In February 2019, Nan Goldin organized groups of people to fill the corkscrew-like halls and drop white pieces of paper meant to look like prescriptions written for

OxyContin (Moynihan, 2019). This was meant to signify the overprescribing that the Purdue company pushed doctors to engage in. The falling of white slips of paper resembled snow falling, in response to Richard Sackler, the son of a Purdue founder, who said years ago that OxyContin's launch would be "followed by a blizzard of prescriptions that will bury the competition" (Sackler in Moynihan 2019, para 4).

As of November 20, 2020, the P.A.I.N. group had circulated a petition with approximately 49,000 signatures with the intent on imposing demands on both the Sackler family and the Purdue Company (Sacklerpain.org). The P.A.I.N. group wants the Purdue Pharma profits and the Sackler money to go to drug treatment facilities, education programs about the dangers associated with opioids, and they want Purdue to fund educational programs to retrain doctors on how to manage pain. They also want the Sackler family to forfeit more of their wealth; at present the family is set to walk away with $12 billion in profits from the sale of drugs manufactured by Purdue including OxyContin (Hopkins and Scurria, 2019).

7.5 PUBLIC COMPANIES INVOLVEMENT AND REACTIONS

Retail pharmacies are being investigated for their role in the opioid crisis. Retail pharmacies are being accused of filling prescriptions when red flags were present. Some accuse retail pharmacies of inadequately training employees on how to report or spot suspicious opioid prescriptions. Ausness (2020) explains some pharmacies improperly trained their employees, did not offer training on how to spot a forged prescription, and structured compensation to reward those who filled the most prescriptions. CVS and Walgreens paid large settlements and claims regarding improper handlings of opioid prescriptions. Ausness (2020) reported CVS agreed to pay $11 million to avoid being charged with violating laws regarding dispensing opioids, CVS agreed to pay a $22 million fine for filling unauthorized prescriptions, and CVS paid $3.5 million to settle a claim involving forged prescriptions. CVS pharmacies in Massachusetts violated the Controlled Substances Act by filling more than 500 forged oxycodone prescriptions. Furthermore, Walgreens was accused of numerous record-keeping and dispensing violations at various dispensing centers and retail stores. Walgreens agreed to pay $80 million to settle and resolve investigations with the Drug Enforcement Agency (Ausness, 2020). Judge Polster ruled in August 2020 that lawsuits against retail pharmacy chains can continue and are a part of the National Prescription Opiate Litigation. The lawsuits claim state retail pharmacies opioid dispensing practices flooded communities with pain pills and were a public nuisance (Gillespie, 2020).

These lawsuits bring up interesting societal questions of responsibility; What is the role of a for-profit pharmacy during the opioid crisis? Walmart, too, has been sued, but Walmart responded a bit different than merely settling the claims for monetary sums. Walmart was accused of not training its employees or enacting policy to monitor suspicious orders before 2011 (Plante, 2019). Walmart has denied wrongdoing. In a legal summary judgment the company stated, "Walmart's distribution accounts for a vanishingly small part of the relevant market: Plaintiffs' own expert concluded that Walmart distributed less than 1.3% of the opioids distributed to two Ohio counties named in the suit. Walmart's motion adds that the company does not market controlled substances and denies culpability in creating a black market for opioids, as alleged by the suit" (Plante, 2019). Walmart responded to the opioid crisis by creating a program, Opioid Stewardship Initiative. In doing so, Walmart abandoned the old model whereby doctors write prescriptions for opioids, and pharmacies fill the prescriptions without asking questions. Walmart is responding to the crisis by implementing strict protocols.

Walmart is taking a comprehensive approach with the Opioid Stewardship Initiative (Kaplan, 2020). First, the company is tackling the issue of fraudulent prescriptions. Beginning January 1, 2020, Walmart will only fill e-prescriptions for opioids and all controlled substances. The rationale for e-prescriptions is two-pronged: e-prescriptions are less prone to errors and are trackable (Kaplan, 2020). The trackable nature of e-prescriptions encourages pharmacies to use NarxCare. "NarxCare is a tool that helps pharmacists make dispensing decisions and provides pharmacists with the real-time interstate visibility that currently exists" ("Walmart's Opioid Stewardship Initiative," 2018, para 3).

Another major component of the initiative is to keep the amounts of opioids prescribed at a low quantity and dosage. One of the most impactful parts of the initiative is that "Walmart and Sam's Club will restrict initial acute opioid prescriptions to no more than a seven-day supply nationwide, with up to a 50-morphine milligram equivalent maximum per day" ("Walmart's Opioid Stewardship Initiative," 2018, para 6). This policy coincides with the CDC guidelines for opioid use, which suggest short-term usage of opioids for acute pain to reduce the likelihood of addiction (CDC, 2018). Walmart is also stocking all of its pharmacies with the drug naloxone, which has life-saving properties for those in the midst of an overdose (Kaplan, 2020). Lastly, Walmart created Dispose Rx which helps with easily disposing left-over opioids, and Walmart remains committed to supporting community education about the dangers of opioids. Pharmacies are not the only businesses taking note of the opioid crisis in the United States. Many other types of businesses are getting involved, and the federal government is encouraging the for-profit sector to offer solutions.

7.6 COMPANIES' RESPONSES TO THE OPIOID CRISIS

Businesses are losing money, decreasing productivity, and paying more for health insurance costs because of the opioid crisis (Davenport et al., 2020) It is not surprising that corporations are doing their part to offer help to those suffering from addiction. Sharing Solutions is a project created in March 2019 by the U.S. Chamber of Commerce to help businesses combat the opioid crisis. Sharing Solutions provides employer resources and showcases all types of creative solutions that companies are implementing. The U.S. Chamber of Commerce and Sharing Solutions believe businesses must be part of the solution and businesses are vehicles to help solve the crisis. Sharing Solutions' staff members traveled to many states hit hard by the opioid crisis including Kentucky, Pennsylvania, Florida, Virginia, Tennessee, and South Carolina and spoke in front of their state's chamber of commerce with community partners to begin the dialogue around business-based solutions in the opioid crisis (U.S. Chamber of Commerce Foundation, 2019).

One of the companies highlighted on the Sharing Solutions website is Leidos, a Fortune 500® information technology, engineering, and science solutions company. An employee of Leidos lost his son to an opioid overdose and the employee shared with the company's CEO his plight and the plight of many others in the company who had lost a family member to opioids or have struggled themselves. In response, CEO Roger Krone launched a series of "education, awareness, and philanthropic relationships to help employees and others prevent—or, if necessary, help treat—addiction" (U.S. Chamber of Commerce Foundation, 2019).

The Leidos corporation took it a step further and created a pledge whereby CEOs acknowledge their role in stopping the opioid crisis and have had numerous other CEOs sign the pledge. The pledge encourages many CEOs to actively participate in ending the crisis. The pledge states,

1. I pledge to help create a workplace where it is safe to have uncomfortable, and often difficult, conversations about addiction.
2. I pledge to help educate my employees about the dangers of prescription opioids, to dispel the myths and stigma surrounding the disease of addiction, and to support employees and family members' access to quality treatment and recovery services.

3. I pledge to support nonprofit organizations dedicated to building drug-free communities and preventing addiction, improving access to quality treatment and supporting recovery.

The Leidos corporation is offering a model for many other companies to follow. The Belden Corporation, also highlighted on the Sharing Solutions website, helps potential employees and current employees construct and implement individual substance abuse counseling and treatment plans the Sharing Solutions project acknowledges the need to explore the connections between the private sector and the public sector.

Connections between the private and the public sector are proving a valuable tool in fighting the opioid crisis. Corporate Socially Responsible (CSR) initiatives described above help strengthen relationships with internal and external stakeholders. Coombs and Holladay (2011) explain stakeholders expect more from companies than to just make a profit, companies now must focus on the Triple Bottom Line. The Triple Bottom line consists of making clear considerations for people, the environment, and profits. People suffering with addiction, and loss of productivity in the workforce, are at the forefront of the CSR initiatives aimed at the opioid crisis. For-profit companies are showing compassion and care for those suffering. Ironically, the opioid crisis was propagated from drug companies only seeking profits, and now the opioid crisis is being lessened in severity by the efforts of for-profit companies.

7.7 INSIDIOUS PRAXIS AND CONCLUSION

Insidious praxis is professional practice that propagates harm and disregards professional ethos. Ultimately, the opioid crisis is a by-product of insidious praxis. Dr. Raymond Sackler, a founder of Purdue Pharma, was enthusiastic during the internal sales rep's visit to his office about the prospects for OxyContin and how it would turn Purdue into a pharmaceutical powerhouse. "OxyContin," he declared, "is our ticket to the moon" (Sackler in Meier, 2018a, p. 41). The crisis began with pharmaceutical CEOs and CMOs looking for a way to increase revenues, and the crisis spread like wildfire after *thought leaders,* doctors who had little regard for rigorous peer-reviewed studies spread the gospel at medical conferences that opioids were the panacea for chronic pain (Lembke, 2016). At these conferences doctors would cite the "landmark Porter and Jick study," yet there was no landmark study; rather Porter and Jick published a short 101-word one-paragraph letter to the editor. The lead author, Hershel Jick, MD, has repeatedly stated that his letter to the editor has been misinterpreted" (Gale, 2016, p. 244). The Porter and Jick letter only discussed short-term opioid use in a hospital setting and did not mention long-term chronic use in a residential setting. Lembke (2016) points out the thought leaders were only chosen by a pharmaceutical company if their work was in support of opioids. The thought leaders' financial arrangements were not made clear to audience members (Lembke, 2016).

These very *thought leaders* were often being paid large sums of money from the pharmaceutical companies, yet they often did not disclose these relationships to the public (Lembke, 2016; Meier, 2018a). Doctors who over-prescribed and knew that their patients were soon addicted yet continued to prescribe is a living manifestation of insidious praxis (Lembke, 2016). Meier (2018a) cites three reasons addiction to opioids occurred: "Some unscrupulous doctors were running 'pill mills,' practices where prescriptions are written without a legitimate purpose in exchange for the price of an office visit. Other doctors were fooled into prescribing the drug to abusers who came in pretending to be patients in pain. People were also forging prescriptions for OxyContin or making duplicate copies of real ones" (p. 14).

Much regret is being expressed in the medical community. One famous thought leader—Russel Portnenoy—admits to lying to other doctors, stating "I gave innumerable lectures in the late 1980s and 1990s about addiction that weren't true," Dr. Portenoy said in a 2010 videotaped interview with a fellow doctor (Catan and Perez, 2012, para 4). The point of this conclusion is not to scapegoat one person or even one company; to the contrary, the point of this conclusion is to highlight the need for a commitment to a professional ethos. Fritz's (2013) work *Professional Civility* stresses professions are homes for the professional, and professionals are entrusted individuals the public seeks out for help and healing. A professional ethos should espouse best practices including citing scholarly peer-reviewed literature, a genuine care for the other, and obligating oneself to first do no harm.

Throughout this book the opioid crisis was explored through the lens of modernity. Modernity is a "risk culture" where risk "becomes fundamental to the way both lay actors and technical specialists organize the social world" (Giddens, 2013, p. 3). The modern world is organized around managing risk (Giddens, 2013, p. 3; Neef, 2012, p. 70). In a way, the opioid crisis is an example of what can happen if risk is mismanaged or if the risks are intentionally distorted. Perdue Pharma and many other major pharmaceutical companies intentionally downplayed the risks of addiction when using opioids for chronic pain (Meier, 2018a). Corporate profits and sales of opioids seemed to trump the risk of addiction to opioids. Pain Societies that were in large part entrusted to educate many physicians about appropriate prescribing were receiving large funds from the pharmaceutical companies (Meier, 2018a, p. 39). Corporate greed and institutional power were promulgating much of this crisis (Meier, 2018a). Large institutions like Joint Commission on Accreditation of Healthcare Organizations, now called the Joint Commission

(JCO), Veterans Health Administration, and the American Pain Society implemented pain as the fifth vital sign. Once the fifth vital sign was implemented, opioids were considered if patients self-reported discomfort of a 4 or greater on a scale of 1–10. This was a pivotal factor in overdispensing of opioids. In modernity, "the primary effect has been to emphasize the values and virtues of instantaneity (instant and fast-food meals, and other satisfactions) and of disposability (cups, plates, cutlery, packaging, napkins, clothing)" (Harvey, 1999, p. 100). Patients wanted their pain to instantly disappear; however, Morris (1998) explains that illness is "situated at the crossroads of biology and culture" (p. 71). The medical community may offer pills before truly understanding the entire cultural-social problem, only treating symptoms, and never touching the main issue.

Modernity promised a commitment to progress; however, some view modernity as "a path paved by fool's gold" (Arnett, 2012, p. 1). Modernity turns away from tradition. If described as a secular religion, the holy trinity of modernity would be progress, efficiency, and individual autonomy (Arnett, 2012, p. 4). In modernity, "the future is constantly drawn into the present by means of the reflexive organization"; reflecting on the past and guiding practices based upon tradition is viewed as unfavorable (Giddens, 2013, p. 3). Narratives of the past in large part were ignored during the opioid crisis. In China during the early nineteenth century there was a societal breakdown as opioids were once seen as a panacea for many ailments. It quickly became obvious that the highly addictive substance led to people dying, families breaking apart as parents were no longer able to care for their children due to addiction, and many becoming imprisoned (Slack, 2001). In the early twentieth century in the United States, opium dens were popping up in America and people would soon become addicted. The U.S. government stepped in and banned opium. In modernity, consumerism pervades culture, with the marketplace at the center, and narratives of the past are dismissed. Many professionals ignored the narratives of the past and focused their attentions on the marketplace and profits.

Understanding framing theory and rhetorical persuasion in modernity is fundamental to studying the crisis. Kuhn's (1970) work is important when examining shifts in the scientific literature. For example, in the 1990s a set of rhetorical facts were constructed to convince doctors that opioids for chronic pain were best practice, but in the early 2000s a new set of rhetorical facts were constructed that opioids were not the best treatment for chronic pain and cause opioid addiction. This book documents the shift from proprescribing literature to conservative opioid prescribing as the prevailing paradigm. This book also documents the different rhetorical biases of pharmaceutical companies, patients, and doctors.

Bibliography

Abraham, N. S., Naik, A. D., & Street, R. L., Jr. (2012). Shared decision making in GI clinic to improve patient adherence. *Clinical Gastroenterology and Hepatology: The Official Clinical Practice Journal of the American Gastroenterological Association*, *10*(8), 825–827. https://doi.org/10.1016/j.cgh.2012.06.001

Agency Medical Directors Group. (2007). *Interagency guideline on opioid dosing for chronic non-cancer pain - wa.* Agency Medical Directors Group. Retrieved May 9, 2022, from https://agencymeddirectors.wa.gov/Files/OpioidGdline.pdf

Ajzen, I. (2012). Martin Fishbein's legacy: The reasoned action approach. *The Annals of the American Academy of Political and Social Science*, *640*, 11–27. www.jstor.org/stable/23218420

Albrecht, T. L., & Goldsmith, D. J. (2003). Social support, social networks, and health. In T. L. Thompson, A. M. Dorsey, K. I. Miller, & R. Parrott (Eds.), *Handbook of health communication* (pp. 263–284). Lawrence Erlbaum Associates Publishers.

Allen, J. A., Duke, J. C., Davis, K. C., Kim, A. E., Nonnemaker, J. M., & Farrelly, M. C. (2015). Using mass media campaigns to reduce youth tobacco use: A review. *American Journal of Health Promotion*, *30*(2), e71–e82. https://doi.org/10.4278/ajhp.130510-LIT-237

American Society of Regional Anesthesia and Pain Medicine. (n.d.). *The specialty of chronic pain management.* www.asra.com/page/44/the-specialty-of-chronic-pain-management.

Anna Lembke. (2017). *Stanford Profiles*, Stanford University. https://profiles.stanford.edu/anna-lembke

Arendt, H. (1963). *Eichmann in Jerusalem*. Penguin.

Arendt, H. (1971). Thinking and moral considerations: A lecture. *Social Research*, *38*(3), 417–446. http://www.jstor.org/stable/40970069

Arendt, H. (2013). *The human condition*. University of Chicago Press.

Aristotle. (2011a). *Aristotle's Nicomachean Ethics* (R. C. Bartlett & S. D. Collins, Trans.). University of Chicago Press.

Aristotle. (2011b). *Rhetoric and poetics*. University of Chicago Press.

Arnett, R. C. (2012). *Communication ethics in dark times: Hannah Arendt's rhetoric of warning and hope*. Southern Illinois University Press.

Arnett, R. C., & A. Holba. (2012). *An overture to philosophy of communication: The carrier of meaning*. Peter Lang.

Arnett, R. C., Harden Fritz, J. M., & Bell, L. M. (2008). *Communication ethics literacy: Dialogue and difference*. Sage Publications.

Ausness, R. C. (2020). Is litigation the way to combat the opioid crisis? *The Journal of Law, Medicine & Ethics*, *48*(2), 293–306. https://doi.org/10.1177/1073110520935341

Bair, M. J., Robinson, R. L., Katon, W., & Kroenke, K. (2003). Depression and pain comorbidity: A literature review. *Archives of Internal Medicine*, *163*(20), 2433–2445. doi:10.1001/archinte.163.20.2433

Ballantyne, J. C. (2007). Regulation of opioid prescribing. *BMJ: British Medical Journal*, *334*(7598), 811–812. www.jstor.org/stable/20506925

Ballantyne, J. C., & Mao, J. (2003). Opioid therapy for chronic pain. *New England Journal of Medicine*, *349*(20), 1943–1953. https://doi .org/10.1056/

Bandura, A., Barbaranelli, C., Caprara, G. V., & Pastorelli, C. (2001). Self-efficacy beliefs as shapers of children's aspirations and career trajectories. *Child Development*, *72*(1), 187–206. www.jstor.org/stable/1132479

Baxter, L. A., & Montgomery, B. M. (1996). *Relating: Dialogues and dialectics*. Guilford Press.

Be Prepared, Be Protected. (2013). iPLEDGE, Isotretinoin REMS: DVD Program Script for Patient Counseling. https://www.fda.gov/media/86293/download#:~:text=IT%20HAS%20ALSO%20BEEN%20REPORTED,CHILDREN%20HAVE%20LOW%20IQ%20SCORES%E2%80%9D.&text=In%20summary%2C%20taking%20isotretinoin%20during,AND%20DISTORTION%20OF%20FACIAL%20STRUCTURE.

Beckman, H. B., Markakis, K. M., Suchman, A. L., & Frankel, R. M. (1994). The doctor-patient relationship and malpractice: Lessons from plaintiff depositions. *Archives of Internal Medicine*, *154*(12), 1365–1370. doi:10.1001/archinte.1994.00420120093010

Bender, K. (2017). Vets adopt alternative treatments for chronic pain after education. *Pain Medicine News*, 1.

Benoit, W. (1995) *Accounts, excuses and apologies: A theory of image repair strategies*. SUNY Press.

Berger, P. L., & Luckmann, T. (1966). *The social construction of reality: A treatise in the sociology of knowledge* (10th ed.). Penguin.

Best, S., & Kellner, D. (1997). *The postmodern turn*. Guilford Press.

Birnbaum, H. G., White, A. G., Schiller, M., Waldman, T., Cleveland, J. M., & Roland, C. L. (2011). Societal costs of prescription opioid abuse, dependence, and misuse in the United States. *Pain Medicine*, *12*(4), 657–667. doi:10.1111/j.1526-4637.2011.01075.x

Bizzell, P., & Herzberg, B. (Eds.). (2001). *The rhetorical tradition: Readings from classical times to the present*. Bedford/St. Martin's Publishing.

Born, M. (2014, Jan.). *3 charged with illegal prescriptions*. Pittsburgh Post-Gazette. https://www.post-gazette.com/local/region/2014/01/17/2-Allegheny-County

-doctors-Westmoreland-County-chiropractor-charged-in-drug-scheme/stories/201401170133

Bowles, J. M., & Lankenau, S. E. (2019). "I gotta go with modern technology, so I'm gonna give 'em the Narcan": The diffusion of innovations and an opioid overdose prevention program. *Qualitative Health Research*, *29*(3), 345–356. https://doi.org/10.1177/1049732318800289

Brandt, A. M. (2007). *The cigarette century: The rise, fall, and deadly persistence of the product that defined America*. Basic Books.

Brain scan may predict best depression treatment. (2013, June 24). National Institutes of Health. www.nih.gov/news-events/nih-research-matters/brain-scan-may-predict-best-depression-treatment

Brennan, M. C., & Rayburn, W. F. (2012). Counseling about risks of congenital anomalies from prescription opioids. *Birth Defects Research Part A: Clinical and Molecular Teratology*, *94*(8), 620–625. https://doi.org/10.1002/bdra.23064

Brookbank, S. (2017, Oct. 6). *Feds: Anderson Township doctor was "fueling opioid epidemic" in Kentucky*. Cincinnati.com. www.cincinnati.com/story/news/2017/10/06/half-million-pills-hundreds-painkiller-feds-anderson-township-doctor-fueling-opioid-epidemic-kentuck/737171001/

Broussard, C. S., Rasmussen, S. A., Reefhuis, J., Friedman, J. M., Jann, M. W., Riehle-Colarusso, T., Honein, M. A., & National Birth Defects Prevention Study. (2011). Maternal treatment with opioid analgesics and risk for birth defects." *American Journal Obstetrics Gynecology*, *204*(4), e311–e314. https://doi.org/10.1016/j.ajog.2010.12.039

Buchwald, E. (2020, March 2). *U.S. health officials say Americans shouldn't wear face masks to prevent CORONAVIRUS—here are 3 other reasons not to wear them*. MarketWatch. https://www.marketwatch.com/story/the-cdc-says-americans-dont-have-to-wear-facemasks-because-of-coronavirus-2020-01-30

Carey, J. (1989). A cultural approach to communication. In *Communication as Culture: Essays on Media and Society*. Unwin Hyman.

Carr, T. M. (2009). *Descartes and the resilience of rhetoric: Varieties of Cartesian rhetorical theory*. Southern Illinois University Press.

Catan, T., & Perez, E. (2012, Dec. 17). A pain-drug champion has second thoughts. *The Wall Street Journal*. www.wsj.com/articles/SB10001424127887324478304578173342657044604

Catan, T., Barrett, D., & Martin, T. W. (2013). Prescription for addiction. In D. Starkman, M. M. Hamilton, R. Chittum, & F. Salmon (Eds.), *The best business writing 2013* (pp. 122–131). Columbia University Press.

Catt, Isaac E. (2012). Communicology and the worldview of antidepressant medicine. *The American Journal of Semiotics*, *28*(1–2), 81–103. https://doi.org/10.5840/ajs2012281-27

Center for Behavioral Health Statistics and Quality. (2016). *2015 national survey on drug use and health: Detailed tables*. Substance Abuse and Mental Health Services Administration.

Centers for Disease Control and Prevention. (2008). Smoking-attributable mortality, years of potential life lose, and productivity losses—United States 2000–2004. *Morbidity and Mortality Weekly Report*, *57*, 1226–1228.

Centers for Disease Control and Prevention. (2016). CDC guideline for prescribing opioids for chronic pain—United States. *Morbidity and Mortality Weekly Report*, *65*(1), 1–49. http://dx.doi.org/10.15585/mmwr.rr6501e1external icon

Centers for Disease Control and Prevention. (2018). *CDC guideline for prescribing opioids for chronic pain*. https://www.cdc.gov/drugoverdose/pdf/prescribing/Guidelines_Factsheet-a.pdf

Centers for Disease Control and Prevention. (2020, May 5). Opioid overdose. https://www.cdc.gov/drugoverdose/index.html

Chou, R., Turner, J. A., Devine, E. B., Hansen, R. N., Sullivan, S. D., Blazina, I., Dana, T., Bougatsos, C., & Deyo, R. A. (2015). The effectiveness and risks of long-term opioid therapy for chronic pain: A systematic review for a National Institutes of Health Pathways to Prevention Workshop. *Annals of Internal Medicine*, *162*(4), 276–286. https://doi.org/10.7326/M14-2559

Cian, L., Krishna, A., & Elder, R. S. (2015). A sign of things to come: Behavioral change through dynamic iconography. *Journal of Consumer Research*, *41*(6), 1426–1446. https://doi.org/10.1086/680673

Cicero, M. T. (1904). *Cicero de oratore: book 1* (E. N. P. Moor, trans.). Methuen.

Cobb, C., Ward, K. D., Maziak, W., Shihadeh, A. L., & Eissenberg, T. (2010). Waterpipe tobacco smoking: An emerging health crisis in the United States. *American Journal of Health Behavior*, *34*(3), 275–285. https://doi.org/10.5993/AJHB.34.3.3

Collier, L. (2018). Young victims of the opioid crisis. *Monitor on Psychology*. www.apa.org/monitor/2018/01/opioid-crisis.aspx

Coombs, W. T., & Holladay, S. J. (2009). *Does what they see affect how they react: Exploring the effects of victim and neutral photographs on reactions to crisis events*. 12th Annual International Public Relations Conference Research That Matters to the Practice, 120–138. Coral Gables, Florida. Accessed May 1, 2022, from http://tinyurl.com/h6zm3hs

Coombs, W. T. (2014). *Ongoing crisis communication: Planning, managing, and responding*. Sage Publications.

Cosio, D., & Lin, E. H. (2015). U.S. veterans increase CAM utilization upon completion of a pain education program. *Alternative Integrated Medicine*, *4*(203). doi:10.4172/2327–5162.1000203

Cosio, D., et al. (2017). *The effects of a pilot functional medicine clinic on chronic pain among veterans*. PAINWeek 2017, September 5–9, Las Vegas, NV.

Costa, A., & Borrowman, M. (2004). Consuming illicit drugs: Disproportionate disadvantage and poor women of color. *ACR Gender and Consumer Behavior*, 7. https://www.acrwebsite.org/volumes/12071/gender/v07/GCB-07

Cottle, S. (2008). Reporting demonstrations: The changing media politics of dissent. *Media, Culture & Society*, *30*(6), 853–872.

Cummings, K. M., & Proctor, R. N. (2014). The changing public image of smoking in the United States: 1964–2014. *Cancer Epidemiology, Biomarkers & Prevention: A*

Publication of the American Association for Cancer Research, Cosponsored by the American Society of Preventive Oncology, *23*(1), 32–36. doi:10.1158/1055-9965. EPI-13–0798

Cunningham, P. W. (2017, Nov. 30). The health 202: Jeff Sessions wants to put more cops on the opioid beat. Experts say that won't solve the problem. *The Washington Post*. www.washingtonpost.com/news/powerpost/paloma/the-health-202/2017/11/30/the-health-202-jeff-sessions-wants-to-put-more-cops-on-the-opioid-beat-experts-say-that-won-t-solve-theproblem/5a1ef05130fb0469e883f90b/?utm_term=.10a65a9f86a7

Cymbalta. (2012, Mar. 14). *Simple pleasures*. AdPharm. adpharm.net/displayimage.php?pid= 34013

Davenport, S., Caverly, M., & Matthews, K. (2020). Economic costs of the opioid crisis for employers. *Benefits Quarterly*, *36*(3), 8–14.

Davis, W. R., & Johnson, B. D. (2008). Prescription opioid use, misuse, and diversion among street drug users in New York City. *Drug and Alcohol Dependence*, *92*(1), 267–276. https://doi.org/10.1016/j.drugalcdep.2007.08.008

Deacon, B. J. (2013). The biomedical model of mental disorder: a critical analysis of its validity, utility, and effects on psychotherapy research. *Clinical Psychology Review*, *33*(7), 846–861. https://doi.org/10.1016/j.cpr.2012.09.007

Desai, R. J., Hernandez-Diaz, S., Bateman, B. T., & Huybrechts, K. F. (2014). Increase in prescription opioid use during pregnancy among Medicaid-enrolled women. *Obstetrics and Gynecology*, *123*(5), 997–1002. https://doi.org/10.1097/AOG.0000000000000208

DeWeerdt, S. (2019, Sept. 11). *Tracing the US opioid crisis to its roots*. Nature. https://www.nature.com/articles/d41586-019-02686-2

Deyo, R. A., Mirza, S. K., Turner, J. A., & Martin, B. I. (2009). Overtreating chronic back pain: Time to back off?" *The Journal of the American Board of Family Medicine*, *22*(1), 62–68. doi:10.3122/jabfm.2009.01.080102

Dostal, R. J. (Ed.). (2002). *The Cambridge companion to Gadamer*. Cambridge University Press.

Dowell, D., Haegerich, T. M., & Chou, R. (2016). CDC guideline for prescribing opioids for chronic pain—United States, 2016. *JAMA*, *315*(15), 1624–1645. doi:10.1001/jama.2016.1464

Drash. (2019, June 24). *Oklahoma judge approves $85 million settlement with opioid drugmaker teva*. https://www.cnn.com/2019/06/24/health/teva-settlement-oklahoma/index.html

Drug Enforcement Agency. (n.d.). *Cannabis, coca, & poppy: Nature's addictive plants*. DEA Museum. https://museum.dea.gov/exhibits/online-exhibits/cannabis-coca-and-poppy-natures-addictive-plants

Dubois, M. Y. (2005). The birth of an ethics charter for pain medicine. *Pain Medicine*, *6*(3), 201–202. https://doi.org/10.1111/j.1526-4637.2005.05046.x

Dutta-Bergman, M. J. (2005). Theory and practice in health communication campaigns: A critical interrogation. *Health Communication*, *18*(2), 103–122. doi:10.1207/s15327027hc1802_1

Dyer, O. (2016). Opioid manufacturer bribed doctors to prescribe fentanyl inappropriately, US says. *BMJ: British Medical Journal (Online)*, 355. https://doi.org/10.1136/bmj.i6742

Ebbeling, C. B., Pawlak, D. B., & Ludwig, D. S. (2002). Childhood obesity: Public-health crisis, common sense cure. *Lancet (London, England)*, *360*(9331), 473–482. https://doi.org/10.1016/S0140-6736(02)09678-2

Eisenberger, N. I. (2012). The pain of social disconnection: Examining the shared neural underpinnings of physical and social pain. *Nature Reviews Neuroscience*, *13*(6), 421. doi:10.1038/nrn3231

Epstein, R., & Street, R. (2011). The values and value of patient-centered care. *The Annals of Family Medicine*, *9*(2), 100–103. doi:10.1370/afm.1239

Eriksen, J., Sjøgren, P., Bruera, E., Ekholm, O., & Rasmussen, N. K. (2006). Critical issues on opioids in chronic non-cancer pain: An epidemiological study. *Pain*, *125*(1–2), 172–179. https://doi.org/10.1016/j.pain.2006.06.009

Erving, G. (1963). *Stigma: Notes on the management of spoiled identity*. Simon & Schuster Inc.

Evans, D. L., Charney, D. S., Lewis, L., Golden, R. N., Gorman, J. M., Krishnan, K. R. R., & Delong, M. R. (2005). Mood disorders in the medically ill: Scientific review and recommendations. *Biological Psychiatry*, *58*(3), 175–189. doi:10.1016/j.biopsych.2005.05.001

Fairhurst, G. T., & Sarr, R. A. (1996). *The art of framing: Managing the language of leadership*. Jossey-Bass Publishers.

Fairhurst, G. T. (2005). Reframing the art of framing: Problems and prospects for leadership. *Leadership*, *1*(2), 165–185. https://doi.org/10.1177/1742715005051857

Fearn-Banks, K. (2010). *Crisis communications: A casebook approach*. Routledge.

Fearn-Banks, K. (2016). *Crisis communications: A casebook approach*. Routledge.

Finch, J. W., Kamien, J. B., & Amass, L. (2007). Two-year experience with buprenorphine-naloxone (Suboxone) for maintenance treatment of opioid dependence within a private practice setting. *Journal of Addiction Medicine*, *1*(2), 104–110. doi:10.1097/ADM.0b013e31809b5df2

Fiore, K. (2016, April 13). *Opioid crisis: Scrap pain as 5th vital sign?* Medical News and Free CME Online. https://www.medpagetoday.com/publichealthpolicy/publichealth/57336

Fisher, W. (1989). *Human communication as narration: Toward a philosophy of reason, value, and action*. University of South Carolina Press.

Foucault, M. (1980). *Power/knowledge: Selected interviews and other writings, 1972–1977*. Pantheon.

Foucault, M. (1982). The subject and power. *Critical Inquiry*, *8*(4), 777–795. http://links.jstor.org/sici?sici=0093-1896%28198222%298%3A4%3C777%3ATSAP%3E2.0.CO%3B2-S

Foucault, M. (2013). *Archaeology of knowledge*. Routledge.

Frankl, V. E. (1985). *Man's search for meaning*. Simon & Schuster.

Frankl, V. E. (2011). *The unheard cry for meaning: Psychotherapy and humanism*. Simon & Schuster.

Franklin, R. (2021, Oct. 9). *Are doctors spending less time with patients?* [web log]. https://mobius.md/2021/10/09/how-much-time-do-physicians-spend-with-patients/

Frieden, T. R., & Houry, D. (2016). Reducing the risks of relief—the CDC opioid-prescribing guideline. *New England Journal of Medicine*, *374*(16), 1501–1504. doi:10.1056/NEJMp1515917

Fritz, J. M. H. (2013). *Professional civility: Communicative virtue at work.* Peter Lang.

Frost, E. A., & Eble, M. F. (Eds.). (2020). *Interrogating gendered pathologies.* University Press of Colorado.

Furlan, A. D., Carnide, N., Irvin, E., Van Eerd, D., Munhall, C., Kim, J., et al. (2018). A systematic review of strategies to improve appropriate use of opioids and to reduce opioid use disorder and deaths from prescription opioids. *Canadian Journal of Pain*, *2*(1), 218–235. doi:10.1080/24740527.2018.1479842

Gadamer, H.-G. (1989). *Truth and method* (J. Weinsheimer & D. G. Marshall, trans.). Continuum.

Gadamer, H.-G. (1996). *The enigma of health: The art of healing in a scientific age.* Polity Press.

Gadamer, H.-G. (2004). *Truth and Method.* Continuum.

Galanti, G.-A. (2014). *Caring for patients from different cultures.* University of Pennsylvania Press.

Gale, A. H. (2016). Drug company compensated physicians role in causing America's deadly opioid epidemic: When will we learn? *Missouri Medicine*, *113*(4), 244–246.

Gallagher, B. K., Shin, Y., & Roohan, P. (2016). Opioid prescriptions among women of reproductive age enrolled in Medicaid—New York, 2008–2013. *Morbidity and Mortality Weekly Report*, *65*(16), 415–417. http://dx.doi.org/10.15585/mmwr.mm6516a2

Giddens, A. (2013). *Modernity and self-identity: Self and society in the late modern age*. John Wiley & Sons.

Giddens, A., & Pierson, C. (1998) *Conversations with Anthony Giddens: Making sense of modernity*. Stanford University Press.

Gillespie, M. (2020, August 8). *Judge rejects bid by CVS, Walgreen's and other pharmacy chains to TOSS opioid suits*. USA Today. https://www.usatoday.com/story/money/business/2020/08/07/cvs-walgreens-other-pharmacies-fail-bid-toss-opioid-lawsuits/3324662001/

Goffman, E. (1963). *Stigma: Notes on the management of spoiled identity*. Simon & Schuster Inc.

Goffman, E. (1974). *Frame analysis: An essay on the organization of experience*. Harvard University Publishing.

Goodnight, G. T. (1982). The personal, technical, and public spheres of argument: A speculative inquiry into the art of public deliberation. *The Journal of the American Forensic Association*, *18*(4), 214–227. doi:10.1080/00028533.1982.11951221

Gourlay, D. L., Heit, H. A., & Almahrezi, A. (2005). Universal precautions in pain medicine: A rational approach to the treatment of chronic pain." *Pain Medicine*, *6*(2), 107–112. https://doi.org/10.1111/j.1526-4637.2005.05031.x

Grassi, E. (2000). *Rhetoric as philosophy: The humanist tradition*. Southern Illinois University Press.

Green, J. (2002). *Babies, blemishes and FDA: A history of Accutane regulation in the United States*. Harvard Library Office for Scholarly Communication. http://nrs.harvard.edu/urn-3:HUL.InstRepos:8963867

Gross, A. G. (2006). *Starring the text: The place of rhetoric in science studies*. Southern Illinois University Press.

Gross, A. G., & Keith, W. M. (1997). *Rhetorical hermeneutics: Invention and interpretation in the age of science*. SUNY Press.

Gross, A. (1990). The origin of species: Evolutionary taxonomy as an example of the rhetoric of science. In H. W. Simons (Ed.), *The Rhetorical Turn: Invention and Persuasion in the Conduct of Inquiry*. University of Chicago Press.

Hackforth, R. (Ed.). (1972). *Plato: Phaedrus* (No. 119). Cambridge University Press.

Haight, S. C., Ko, J. Y., Tong, V. T., Bohm, M. K., & Callaghan, W. M. (2018). Opioid use disorder documented at delivery hospitalization—United States, 1999–2014. *Morbidity and Mortality Weekly Report*, *67*(31), 845. doi:10.15585/mmwr.mm6731a1

Hairston, M. (1982). The winds of change: Thomas Kuhn and the revolution in the teaching of writing. *College Composition and Communication*, *33*(1), 76–88. https://doi.org/10.2307/357846

Hall, J. A., Horgan, T. G., Stein, T. S., & Roter, D. L. (2002). Liking in the physician–patient relationship. *Patient Education and Counseling*, *48*(1), 69–77.

Hall, S. (2001). Foucault: Power, knowledge and discourse. In M. Wetherell, S. Taylor, & S. J. Yates (Eds.), *Discourse Theory and Practice: A Reader* (pp. 72–81). Sage Publications.

Hals, T. (2019, Dec. 4). *U.S. regions hard hit by opioids to ditch class action, pursue own lawsuits*. https://www.reuters.com/article/us-usa-opioids-litigation/u-s-regions-hard-hit-by-opioids-to-ditch-class-action-pursue-own-lawsuits-idUSKBN1Y72C6

Hartelius, E. J. (2012). Revisiting Vico's pedagogy of invention: The intellectual entrepreneurship pre-graduate school internship." *Quarterly Journal of Speech*, *98*(2), 153–177. doi:10.1080/00335630.2012.66349

Harvey, D. (1999). Time-space compression and the postmodern condition. In M. Waters (Ed.), *Modernity: Critical Concepts, Volume IV, After Modernity* (pp. 98–118). Routledge.

Hearit, K. M. (2006). *Crisis management by apology: Corporate response to allegations of wrongdoing*. Routledge.

Hernández, L. H., & Dean, M. (2020). I felt very discounted. In E. A. Frost & M. F. Eble (Eds.), *Interrogating Gendered Pathologies*. University Press of Colorado.

Herrick, J. A. (2001). *The history of rhetoric: An introduction*. Allyn and Bacon.

Hilden, D. (2018, Mar. 9). *Opioids for back, knee, and hip pain? A chat with Dr. Erin Krebs*. Health and Wellness by Dr. David Hilden, myhealthymatters.org/opioids-for-back-knee-and-hip-pain-a-chat-with-dr-erin-krebs/

Hoffman, J. (2019, Aug. 26). *Johnson & Johnson ordered to pay $572 million in landmark opioid trial*. https://www.nytimes.com/2019/08/26/health/oklahoma-opioids-johnson-and-johnson.html

Holton, R. (2016). Addiction, self-signaling and the deep self. *Mind & Language, 31*(3), 300–313. doi:10.1111/mila.12107

Holzman, D. (2018, Feb. 21). *Insurance status, physician input affect outcomes on prenatal care in opioid-dependent mothers.* Pain Medicine News. www.painmedicinenews.com/Clinical-Pain-Medicine/Article/12-17/Insurance-Status-Physician-Input-Affect-Outcomes-on-Prenatal-Care-in-Opioid-Dependent-Mothers/46890

Hopkins, J. S., & Scurria, A. (2019, Oct. 5). *Sacklers received as much as $13 billion in profits from Purdue Pharma.* The Wall Street Journal. https://www.wsj.com/articles/sacklers-received-12-billion-to-13-billion-in-profits-from-oxycontin-maker-purdue-pharma-11570221797

Houk, Vernon N., et al. (1992) Recommendations for the use of folic acid to reduce the number of cases of spina bifida and other neural tube defects." *MMWR. Recommendations and Reports: Morbidity and Mortality Weekly Report. Recommendations and Reports/Centers for Disease Control, 41*(14), 1–7.

Inciardi, J. A., Surratt, H. L., Kurtz, S. P., & Cicero, T. J. (2007). Mechanisms of prescription drug diversion among drug-involved club- and street-based populations. *Pain Medicine, 8*(2), 171–183.

Inturrisi, C. E. (2002). Clinical pharmacology of opioids for pain. *The Clinical Journal of Pain, 18*(4 Suppl), S3–S13. https://doi.org/10.1097/00002508-200207001-00002

iPledge Program. (2016). *iPledge committed to pregnancy prevention.* https://www.ipledgeprogram.com/iPledgeUI/rems/pdf/resources/The%20iPLEDGE%20Program%20Patient%20Introductory%20Brochure.pdf

Ivie, R. L. (2015). Enabling democratic dissent. *Quarterly Journal of Speech, 101*(1), 46–59. doi:10.1080/00335630.2015.994900

Jackson, J. E. (2000). Me/not-me: Self, language, and pain. In *"Camp pain": Talking with chronic pain patients* (pp. 143–168). University of Pennsylvania Press.

Jansson, L. M., Velez, M., & Harrow, C. (2009). The opioid exposed newborn: Assessment and pharmacologic management. *Journal of Opioid Management, 5*(1), 47.

Janz, N. K., & Becker, M. H. (1984). The health belief model: A decade later. *Health Education Quarterly, 11*(1), 1–47. https://doi.org/10.1177/109019818401100101

Kaplan, R. (2020). Walmart's opioid stewardship initiative rhetorically constructed as an act of corporate social responsibility. *Speaker & Gavel, 57*(1), 5.

Kattan, J. A., Tuazon, E., Paone, D., Dowell, D., Vo, L., Starrels, J. L., Jones, C. M., & Kunins, H. V. (2016). Public health detailing: A successful strategy to promote judicious opioid analgesic prescribing. *American Journal of Public Health, 106*(8), 1430–1438. https://doi.org/10.2105/AJPH.2016.303274

Keefe, P. R. (2017). The family that built an empire of pain. *The New Yorker, 30.*

Kelley, M. S., Su, D., & Britigan, D. H. (2016). Disparities in health information access: Results of a county-wide survey and implications for health communication. *Health Communication, 31*(5), 575–582. https://doi.org/10.1080/10410236.2014.979976

Kimball, B. A. (1996). *The "true professional ideal" in America: A history.* Rowman & Littlefield.

Kissin, I. (2013). Long-term opioid treatment of chronic nonmalignant pain: Unproven efficacy and neglected safety? *Journal of Pain Research*, *6*, 513. 10.2147/JPR.S47182

Kleinfield, N. R. (2012, Jan. 11). *Oxycodone prescriptions rose sharply in New York*. New York Times. http://www.nytimes.com/2012/01/12/nyregion/oxycodone-prescriptions-rose-sharply-in-new-york-schneidermanreport-says.html?ref=prescriptiondrugabuse

Kocherlakota P. (2014). Neonatal abstinence syndrome. *Pediatrics*, *134*(2), e547–e561. https://doi.org/10.1542/peds.2013-3524

Kodjak, Alison. (2016, July 6). *Obama administration eases restrictions on doctors who treat opioid addiction*. NPR. www.npr.org/sections/healthshots/2016/07/06/484843560/obama-administration-eases-restrictions-on-doctors-who-treat-opioid-addiction

Kolesar, T. (2017, June 23). *Centre county physician arrested for prescribing opioid pain pills outside his practice*. The Progress. www.theprogressnews.com/centre-county-physician-arrested-for-prescribing-opioid-pain-pills-outside/article_5b3bfb2d-7f25-5e23-bd05-48442dee9a68.html

Koob, G. F. (2000). Neurobiology of addiction: Toward the development of new therapies. *Annals of the New York Academy of Sciences*, 909, 170–185. doi:10.1111/j.1749-6632.2000.tb06682.x

Korsch, B. M. (2011). Forward. In T. L. Thompson (Ed.)., *The Routledge Handbook of Health Communication*. Routledge.

Koschmann, T. (Ed.). (1996). Paradigm shifts and instructional technology: An introduction. In *CSCL: Theory and Practice of an Emerging Paradigm* (pp. 1–23). Routledge.

Kosten, T. R., & Haile, C. N. (2014). Opioid-related disorders. Kasper D, & Fauci A, & Hauser S, & Longo D, & Jameson J, & Loscalzo J. (Eds.), *Harrison's Principles of Internal Medicine* (19th ed.). McGraw Hill. https://accessmedicine.mhmedical.com/content.aspx?bookid=1130&sectionid=79757372

Kovacs, R. J., Gilbert, J. H., & Oetgen, W. J. (2020). Call to action: Opioid crisis impacting more than just patients. *Journal of the American College of Cardiology*, *75*(3), 341–343. https://doi.org/10.1016/j.jacc.2019.12.010

Kraft W. K., Stover, M. W., & Davis, J. M. (2016). Neonatal abstinence syndrome: Pharmacologic strategies for the mother and infant. *Seminars in Perinatology*, *40*(3), 203–212. doi:10.1053/j.semperi.2015.12.007

Kuhn, T. S. (1970). *The structure of scientific revolutions* (2nd ed.). University of Chicago Press.

Kutner, M., Greenberg, E., Jin, Y., & Paulsen, C. (2006). The health literacy of America's adults: Results from the 2003 National Assessment of Adult Literacy. NCES 2006–483. *National Center for Education Statistics*.

Lembke, A. (2016). *Drug dealer, MD: How doctors were duped, patients got hooked, and why it's so hard to stop*. John Hopkins University Press.

Littlefield, R. S., & Sellnow, T. L. (2015). *Risk and crisis communication: Navigating the tensions between organizations and the public*. Lexington Books.

Lopez, G. (2017, June 6). *In one year, drug overdoses killed more Americans than the entire Vietnam war did.* Vox. www.vox.com/policy-and-politics/2017/6/6/15743986/opioid-epidemic-overdose-deaths-2016

Luoma, J. B., Twohig, M. P., Waltz, T., Hayes, S. C., Roget, N., Padilla, M., & Fisher, G. (2007). An investigation of stigma in individuals receiving treatment for substance abuse. *Addictive Behaviors, 32*(7), 1331–1346. https://doi.org/10.1016/j.addbeh.2006.09.008

Lyotard, J.-F. (1993). Excerpts from *The Postmodern Condition: A Report on Knowledge*. In J. Natoli & L. Hutchcon (Eds.), *A Postmodern Reader* (pp. 71–90). SUNY Press.

Magee, G. A. (2010). *The Hegel dictionary*. Continuum.

Mager, R. (1972). *Goal analysis*. Fearon Publishers.

Manchikanti, L. (2007). National drug control policy and prescription drug abuse: Facts and fallacies." *Pain Physician, 10*(3), 399.

Mann, B. (2020, July 17). *Doctors and dentists still flooding U.S. with opioid prescriptions*. NPR. https://www.npr.org/2020/07/17/887590699/doctors-and-dentists-still-flooding-u-s-with-opioid-prescriptions

Martin, S. (2012). *Opium fiend: A 21st century slave to a 19th century addiction.* Random House Inc.

May, S., & Mumby, D. K. (Eds.). (2005). *Engaging organizational communication theory and research: Multiple perspectives*. Sage.

Meier, B. (2018a). *Pain killer: An empire of deceit and the origin of America's opioid epidemic*. Random House.

Meier, B. (2018b, June 8). *Every time I thought the Purdue Pharma OxyContin story was over, I was wrong*. The New York Times. www.nytimes.com/2018/06/08/insider/i-thought-the-purdue-pharma-oxycontin-story-was-over-i-was-wrong.html

Meldrum M. L. (2016). The ongoing opioid prescription epidemic: Historical context. *American Journal of Public Health, 106*(8), 1365–1366. https://doi.org/10.2105/AJPH.2016.303297

Melzak, R. (1999). From the gate to the Neuromatrix. *Pain* (Supplement 6), S121–S126. doi:10.1016/S0304-3959(99)00145–1

Mikeladze, G., Thirtyacre, J., Norman, S., Kraus, C., & Huynh, C. (n.d.). *Chronic pain management program*. Kaiser Permanente. https://mydoctor.kaiserpermanente.org/ncal/Images/CP_Brochure_01.11.16_tcm75-1140673.pdf

Miles, S. H. (2005). *The Hippocratic oath and the ethics of medicine*. Oxford University Press.

Moghe, S. (2016, Oct. 14). *Opioids: From "wonder drug" to abuse epidemic*. CNN. www.cnn.com/2016/05/12/health/opioid-addiction-history/index.html

Morone, N. E., & Weiner, D. K. (2013). Pain as the fifth vital sign: Exposing the vital need for pain education. *Clinical Therapeutics, 35*(11), 1728–1732. https://doi.org/10.1016/j.clinthera.2013.10.001

Morrell, A. (2016, March 24). The oxycontin clan: The $14 Billion newcomer to forbes 2015 list of richest U.S. families. *Forbes*. Retrieved May 9, 2022, from https://www.forbes.com/sites/alexmorrell/2015/07/01/the-oxycontin-clan-the-14-billion-newcomer-to-forbes-2015-list-of-richest-u-s-families/?sh=7f14e41475e0

Morris, D. B. (1991). *The culture of pain*. University of California Press.

Morris, D. B. (1998). *Illness and culture in the postmodern age*. University of California Press.

Moss, G. E. (1973). *Illness, immunity, and social interaction: The dynamics of biosocial resonation*. Wiley.

Moynihan, C. (2019, Feb. 10). *Guggenheim targeted by protesters for accepting money from family with OxyContin ties*. The New York Times. https://www.nytimes.com/2019/02/09/arts/protesters-guggenheim-sackler.html

Mularski, R. A., White-Chu, F., Overbay, D., Miller, L., Asch, S. M., & Ganzini, L. (2006). Measuring pain as the 5th vital sign does not improve quality of pain management. *Journal of General Internal Medicine*, *21*(6), pp. 607–612. doi:10.1111/j.1525-1497.2006.00415.x

National Alliance of Advocates for Buprenorphine Treatment. (2018). *What exactly is buprenorphine?* The National Alliance of Advocates for Buprenorphine Treatment. www.naabt.org/faq_answers.cfm?ID=2.kickbacks.html?partner=rss&emc=rss

National Institute on Drug Abuse. (2014, July 1). *Drugs, brains, and behavior: The science of addiction*. https://www.drugabuse.gov/publications/drugs-brains-behavior-science-addiction

National Prescription Opiate Litigation. (2020). No. 19–4099 (6th Cir. 2020). http://bristolvt.org/wp-content/uploads/2019/10/VI_Northern_Ohio_US_District_Court_Opiods_Class_Action_Suit_notice_2019-09-11.pdf

Neef, D. (2012), *Managing corporate reputation and risk*. Routledge.

Okie, S. (2010). A flood of opioids, a rising tide of deaths. *New England Journal of Medicine*, *363*(21), 1981–1985. doi:10.1056/NEJMp1011512

Olawepo, J. O., Pharr, J. R., & Kachen, A. (2019). The use of social marketing campaigns to increase HIV testing uptake: A systematic review. *AIDS Care*, *31*(2), 153–162. doi:10.1080/09540121.2018.1533631

Olsen, Y., & Sharfstein, J. M. (2014). Confronting the stigma of opioid use disorder—and its treatment. *JAMA*, *311*(14), 1393–1394. doi:10.1001/jama.2014.2147

Opioids for chronic pain: Addiction is not rare. (2011, Oct. 30). YouTube, uploaded by Andrew Kolodny. https://www.youtube.com/watch?v=DgyuBWN9D4w

P.A.I.N. Sackler. (2018). https://www.sacklerpain.org/

Pan, P.-L., & Meng, J. (2016, June). Media frames across stages of health crisis: A crisis management approach to news coverage of flu pandemic. *Journal of Contingencies & Crisis Management*, *24*(2), 95–106.

Patrick, S. W., Schumacher, R. E., Benneyworth, B. D., Krans, E. E., McAllister, J. M., & Davis, M. M. (2012). Neonatal abstinence syndrome and associated health care expenditures: United States, 2000–2009. *JAMA*, *207*(18), 1934–1940. doi:10.1001/jama.2012.3951

Pecchioni, L. L., & Keeley, M. P. (2011). Insights about health from family communication theories. In T. L. Thompson, A. R. Parrott, & J. Nussbaum (Eds.), *Routledge Handbook of Health Communication* (pp. 363–376). Routledge.

Pechmann, C. (2001). A comparison of health communication models: Risk learning versus stereotype priming. *Media Psychology, 3*(2), 189–210. https://doi.org/10.1207/S1532785XMEP0302_04

Penm, J., MacKinnon, N. J., Boone, J. M., Ciaccia, A., McNamee, C., & Winstanley, E. L. (2017). Strategies and policies to address the opioid epidemic: A case study of Ohio. *Journal of the American Pharmacists Association, 57*(2S), S148–S153. https://doi.org/10.1016/j.japh.2017.01.001

Perez-Pena, R. (2017, May 31). *Ohio sues drug makers, saying they aided opioid epidemic*. The New York Times. www.nytimes.com/2017/05/31/us/ohio-sues-pharmaceutical-drug-opioid-epidemic-mike-dewine.html

Perlstein, M. (1947). Congenital morphinism: A rare cause of convulsions in the newborn. *JAMA, 135*(10), 633. doi:10.1001/jama.1947.62890100006006c

Pernot, L. (2005). *Rhetoric in antiquity*. Catholic University America Press.

Physicians for Responsible Opioid Prescribing. (2016a, April 13). Letter to Mark Chassin, MD, MPH president and CEO The Joint Commission. http://www.supportprop.org/wp-content/uploads/2014/12/TJC-Letter-Final-04-11-16.pdf

Physicians for Responsible Opioid Prescribing. (2016b, April 13). Citizen petition to the Centers for Medicare and Medicaid Services (CMS) requesting changes to the HCAHPS survey. Received by Andy Slavitt, Acting Administrator Centers, for Medicare & Medicaid Services.

Pickard, H. (2016). Denial in addiction. *Mind & Language, 31*(3), 277–299. doi:10.1111/mila.12106

Plante, S. (2019, July 23). *Walmart and CVS are among the retailers being sued for aiding the spread of opioids*. https://www.vox.com/the-goods/2019/7/23/20707179/walmart-cvs-walgreens-opioid-crisis-lawsuit-trial

Plato. (380 BCE). *Gorgias* (B. Jowett, trans.). The Internet Classics Archive. classics.mit.edu/Plato/gorgias.html

Platt, C. (2014). *King death: The Black Death and its aftermath in late-medieval England*. Routledge.

Podolsky, S. H. (2015). *The antibiotic era: Reform, resistance, and the pursuit of a rational therapeutics*. JHU Press.

Podolsky, S. H., Herzberg, D., & Greene, J. A. (2019). Preying on prescribers (and their patients)—Pharmaceutical marketing, iatrogenic epidemics, and the Sackler legacy. *New England Journal of Medicine, 380*(19), 1785–1787.

Polster, J. (2019, September 26). *United States District court northern district of Ohio Eastern division*. https://www.ohnd.uscourts.gov/sites/ohnd/files/2676.pdf

Portenoy, R. K., & Foley, K. M. (1986). Chronic use of opioid analgesics in non-malignant pain: Report of 38 cases. *Pain, 25*(2), 171–186. doi:10.1016/0304-3959(86)90091–6

Posner, G., & Brubaker, R. (2020, July 22). *The Sacklers could get away with it*. The New York Times. https://www.nytimes.com/2020/07/22/opinion/sacklers-opioid-epidemic.html

Purdue Pharma OxyContin commercial. (2016, Sept. 22). YouTube. www.youtube.com/watch?v=Er78Dj5hyeI

Rainville, J., Hartigan, C., Martinez, E., Limke, J., Jouve, C., & Finno, M. (2004). Exercise as a treatment for chronic low back pain. *The Spine Journal*, *4*(1), 106–115. doi:10.1016/s1529-9430(03)00174–8

Rasyidi, E., Wilkins, J. N., & Danovitch, I. (2012). Training the next generation of providers in addiction medicine. *Psychiatric Clinics of North America*, *35*(2), 461–480. https://doi.org/10.1016/j.psc.2012.04.001

Raymond, N. (2019, March 26). *Purdue pharma agrees to $270 million settlement in Oklahoma opioid case*. https://www.reuters.com/article/us-usa-opioids-litigation/oxycontin-maker-purdue-agrees-to-settle-oklahoma-opioid-case-source-idUSKCN1R70CH

Recommendations for the use of folic acid to reduce the number of cases of spina bifida and other neural tube defects. (1992). *MMWR*, *41*(14), 1–7.

Redsand, A. (2006). *Viktor Frankl: A life worth living*. Houghton Mifflin Harcourt.

Renthal, W. (2016). Seeking balance between pain relief and safety: CDC issues new opioid-prescribing guidelines. *JAMA Neurology*, *73*(5), 513–514. doi:10.1001/jamaneurol.2016.0535

Rettie, R. (2004, Oct.). Using Goffman's frameworks to explain presence and reality. In *7th Annual International Workshop on Presence*, Valencia, Spain (pp. 117–124).

Rimal, R. N., & Lapinski, M. K. (2009). Why health communication is important in public health. *Bulletin of the World Health Organization*, *87*(4), 247–247a. doi:10.2471/BLT.08.056713

Ritchie, A. J. (2017). *Invisible no more: Police violence against Black women and women of color*. Beacon Press.

Roberts, H. A., & Veil, S. R. (2015). The tension of emotional connection. In R. Littlefield & T. L. Sellnow (Eds.), *Risk and Crisis Communication: Navigating the Tensions between Organizations and the Public* (pp. 123–139). Lexington Books.

Roberts, W. R. (trans.). (1954). *Aristotle: Rhetoric and poetics*. The Modern Library.

Rogers, E. M. (1983). *Diffusion of innovations* (3rd ed.). New York.

Rose, M. (2018). Are prescription opioids driving the opioid crisis? Assumptions vs facts. *Pain Medicine*, *19*(4), 793–807. https://doi.org/10.1093/pm/pnx048

Rosenberg, T. (2007). When is a pain doctor a drug pusher? *New York Times Magazine*.

Ross, D. (2009). *Introduction. The Nicomachean Ethics, by Aristotle*. Oxford University Press.

Rossman-McKinney, K. (2019). *Michigan goes after OPIOID distributors, files lawsuit under Michigan drug DEALER Liability Act*. https://www.michigan.gov/ag/0,4534,7-359-92297_92299-514835--,00.html

Roter, D. L., & Hall, J. A. (2004). Physician gender and patient-centered communication: A critical review of empirical research. *Annual Review Public Health*, *25*, 497–519. https://doi.org/10.1146/annurev.publhealth.25.101802.123134

Rudd, R. A., Seth, P., David, F., & Scholl, L. (2016). Increases in drug and opioid overdose deaths—United States, 2000–2014." *American Journal of Transplantation*, *16*(4), 1323–1327. http://onlinelibrary.wiley.com/doi/10.1111/ajt.13776/full

Russeth, A. (2019, Nov. 18). *Nan Goldin, P.A.I.N. group stage protest against Sackler family, Purdue Pharmaceuticals in Met's Sackler wing*. ARTnews.com. https://www.artnews.com/art-news/news/nan-goldin-p-n-group-stage-protest-sackler-family-purdue-pharmaceuticals-mets-sackler-wing-9946/

Sales, B. (2019, May 22). *Who are the SACKLERS, the family at the center of the OPIOID crisis?* https://www.jta.org/2019/05/22/united-states/who-are-the-sacklers-the-family-at-the-center-of-the-opioid-crisis

Sarin, I. (2009). *The global vision: Karl Jaspers*. Peter Lang.

Savage, S. R., Joranson, D. E., Covington, E. C., Schnoll, S. H., Heit, H. A., & Gilson, A. M. (2003). Definitions related to the medical use of opioids: Evolution towards universal agreement. *Journal of Pain and Symptom Management*, *26*(1), 655–667. https://doi.org/10.1016/S0885-3924(03)00219-7

Savage, T. (2017, July 5). *Painful pills: Oklahoma sues opioid producers*. https://nondoc.com/2017/06/30/oklahoma-lawsuit-opioid-producers/

Schiavo, R. (2013). *Health communication: From theory to practice*. John Wiley & Sons.

Schrag, C. O. (1999). *The self after postmodernity*. Yale University Press.

Scott, K. M., Bruffaerts, R., Tsang, A., Ormel, J., Alonso, J., Angermeyer, M. C., Benjet, C., Bromet, E., de Girolamo, G., de Graaf, R., Gasquet, I., Gureje, O., Haro, J. M., He, Y., Kessler, R. C., Levinson, D., Mneimneh, Z. N., Oakley Browne, M. A., Posada-Villa, J., Stein, D. J., Takeshima, T., & Von Korff, M. (2007). Depression–anxiety relationships with chronic physical conditions: Results from the World Mental Health Surveys. *Journal of Affective Disorders*, *103*(1), 113–120. https://doi.org/10.1016/j.jad.2007.01.015

Sellnow, T. L., & Seeger, M. W. (2013). *Theorizing crisis communication*. Volume 4. John Wiley & Sons.

Sim, S. (Ed.). (2001). *The Routledge companion to postmodernism*. Routledge.

Slack, E. R. (2001). The effects of opium on Chinese society. In *Opium, state and society: China's narco-economy and the Guomindang, 1924–1937* (pp. 34–62). University of Hawaii Press.

Smith, F. (2017, Oct.). *Babies fall victim to the opioid crisis*. National Geographic. www.nationalgeographic.com/magazine/2017/09/science-of-addiction-babies-opioids/

Smith, S. (2014). *New pain pill's approval: "Genuinely frightening."* CNN.com/2014/02/26/health/zohydro-approval/index.html

Street Jr, R. L., Makoul, G., Arora, N. K., & Epstein, R. M. (2009). How does communication heal? Pathways linking clinician–patient communication to health outcomes. *Patient Education and Counseling*, *74*(3), 295–301. https://doi.org/10.1016/j.pec.2008.11.015

Street, R. L., Jr. (2003). Communication in medical encounters: An ecological perspective. In T. L. Thompson, A. M. Dorsey, K. I. Miller, & R. Parrott (Eds.), *Handbook of health communication* (pp. 63–89). Lawrence Erlbaum Associates Publishers.

Stuart, H. (2019, March). Managing the stigma of opioid use. *Healthcare Management Forum*, *32*(2), 78–83. https://doi.org/10.1177/0840470418798658

Sturgeon, J. A., & Zautra, A. J. (2016). Social pain and physical pain: Shared paths to resilience. *Pain Management*, *6*(1), 63–74. https://doi.org/10.2217/pmt.15.56

Sullivan, M. J., & D'Eon, J. L. (1990). Relation between catastrophizing and depression in chronic pain patients. *Journal of Abnormal Psychology*, *99*(3), 260–263. https://doi.org/10.1037/0021-843X.99.3.260

Sutton, M. Y., Jones, R. L., Wolitski, R. J., Cleveland, J. C., Dean, H. D., & Fenton, K. A. (2009). A review of the Centers for Disease Control and Prevention's response to the HIV/AIDS crisis among blacks in the United States, 1981–2009. *American Journal of Public Health, 99*(S2), S351–S359.

Tavernise, S. (2011). "Ohio County losing its young to painkillers' grip." *The New York Times*, 1.

The American Cancer Society Medical and Editorial Content Team. (2019). Facts about cancer pain. www.cancer.org/treatment/treatments-and-side-effects/physical-side-effects/pain/facts-about-cancer-pain.html

Thompson, T. L., Parrott, R., & Nussbaum, J. F. (Eds.). (2003). *Handbook of health communication*. Routledge.

Thompson, T. L., Parrott, R., & Nussbaum, J. F. (Eds.). (2011). *The Routledge handbook of health communication* (2nd ed.). Routledge.

Todman, D. (2007). Childbirth in ancient Rome: From traditional folklore to obstetrics. *Australian and New Zealand Journal of Obstetrics and Gynecology*, *47*(2), 82–85. https://doi.org/10.1111/j.1479-828X.2007.00691.x

Tolia, V. N., Patrick, S. W., Bennett, M. M., Murthy, K., Sousa, J., Smith, P. B., Clark, R. H., & Spitzer, A. R. (2015). Increasing incidence of the neonatal abstinence syndrome in US neonatal ICUs. *New England Journal of Medicine*, *372*(22), 2118–2126. doi:10.1056/NEJMsa1500439

Tosches, N. (2002). *The last opium den*. Bloomsbury Publishing USA.

Tulke, J. (2020). Archiving dissent: (Im)material trajectories of political street art in Istanbul and Athens. In A. McGarry, I. Erhart, H. Eslen-Ziya, O. Jenzen, & U. Korkut (Eds.), *The aesthetics of global protest: Visual culture and communication* (pp. 121–140). Amsterdam University Press.

Turk, D. C., & Okifuji, A. (2002). Psychological factors in chronic pain: Evolution and revolution. *Journal of Consulting and Clinical Psychology*, *70*(3), 678–690. https://doi.org/10.1037/0022-006X.70.3.678

"Two innovative approaches for treating opioid addiction." (2018, Sept. 5). *Blue Cross Blue Shield Association*. www.bcbs.com/the-health-of-america/articles/two-innovative-approaches-treating-opioid-addiction

Tyson, P. (2001). The Hippocratic oath today. *Nova, 21*.

Understanding pain. (2016, July 26). Mayo Clinic, Mayo Foundation for Medical Education and Research. www.mayoclinic.org/understanding-pain/art-20208632

U.S. Attorney's Office. (2017, Dec. 12). *Elko cardiologist arrested on opioid and fraud charges*. KOLO. www.kolotv.com/content/news/Elko-cardiologist-arrested-on-opioid-and-fraud-charges-463702723.html

U.S. Chamber of Commerce Foundation. (2019). *Sharing Solutions Businesses Combat the Opioid Crisis. Sharing Solutions*. Retrieved May 11, 2022, from https://sharingsolutions.us/

U.S. Department of Health and Human Services & Centers for Disease Control and Prevention. Office of the Surgeon General Murthy. (2016, Nov.). *Facing addiction in America: The Surgeon General's report on alcohol, drugs and health*. U.S. Department of Health and Human Services.

U.S. Department of Health and Human Services. (2018, Jan. 16). *Development & approval process (drugs)*. US Food and Drug Administration.

U.S. Department of Health and Human Services & Centers for Disease Control and Prevention. (2008). Smoking-attributable mortality, years of potential life lost, and productivity losses—United States, 2000–2004. *Morbidity and Mortality Weekly Report*, *57*(45), 1226.

U.S. Department of Health and Human Services & Centers for Disease Control and Prevention. (2011, Nov. 4). Vital signs: Overdoses of prescription opioid pain relievers—United States, 1999–2008. *Morbidity and Mortality Weekly Report*, *60*(43), 1–6.

U.S. Department of Health and Human Services & Centers for Disease Control and Prevention. (2017, Jan. 11). Healthy people. Centers for Disease Control and Prevention. www.cdc.gov/nchs/healthy_people/index.htm

U.S. Department of Health and Human Services & U.S. Food and Drug Administration. (n.d.). *Approved risk evaluation and mitigation strategies (REMS)*. www.accessdata.fda.gov/scripts/cder/rems/index.cfm

U.S. Department of Health and Human Services, National Institutes of Health, & National Institute on Drug Abuse. (2015, Sept. 1). Dramatic increases in maternal opioid use and neonatal abstinence syndrome. www.drugabuse.gov/related-topics/trends-statistics/infographics/dramatic-increases-in-maternal-opioid-use-neonatal-abstinence-syndrome

U.S. Department of Health, Education and Welfare, Public Health Service Publication. (1964). *Report of the Advisory Committee to the Surgeon General of the Public Health Service*. No. 1103.

U.S. General Accounting Office. (2003). *Prescription drugs OxyContin abuse and diversion and efforts to address the problem*. U.S. General Accounting Office.

Van Ree, J. M., Gerrits, M. A. F. M., & Vanderschuren, L. J. M. J. (1999). Opioids, reward and addiction: An encounter of biology, psychology, and medicine. *Pharmacological Reviews*, *51*(2), 341–396.

Van Way, C. W. (2019). Bashing big pharma. *Missouri Medicine*, *116*(2), 80–82.

Vasaly, A. (1996). *Representations: Images of the world in ciceronian oratory*. University of California Press.

Verene, D. P. (1981). *Vico's science of imagination*. Cornell University Press.

Vestal, C. (2019, Feb. 14). *Pay attention to this little-noticed opioid lawsuit in Oklahoma*. https://www.pewtrusts.org/en/research-and-analysis/blogs/stateline/2019/02/14/pay-attention-to-this-little-noticed-opioid-lawsuit-in-oklahoma

Vico, G. (1990). *On the study methods of our time*. Cornell University Press.

Viswanath, K. (2006). Public communications and its role in reducing and eliminating health disparities. In *Examining the health disparities research plan of the National Institutes of Health: Unfinished business* (pp. 215–253). Institute of Medicine.

Volkow, N. D., & Collins, F. S. (2017). The role of science in addressing the opioid crisis. *New England Journal of Medicine, 377*(4), 391–394. doi:10.1056/NEJMsr1706626

Volkow, N. D., & McLellan, A. T. (2016). Opioid abuse in chronic pain—misconceptions and mitigation strategies. *New England Journal of Medicine, 374*(13), 1253–1263. doi:10.1056/NEJMra1507771

Wachholtz A. B., Pearce, M. J., & Koenig, H. (2007). Exploring the relationship between spirituality, coping, and pain." *Journal of Behavioral Medicine, 30*, 311–318.

Wachholtz A. B., Gonzalez, G., Boyer, E., Naqvi, Z. N., Rosenbaum, C., & Ziedonis, D. (2011). Intersection of chronic pain treatment and opioid analgesic misuse: Causes, treatments, and policy strategies. *Substance Abuse and Rehabilitation, 2*, 145.

Wagner, K. D., Oman, R. F., Smith, K. P., Harding, R. W., Dawkins, A. D., Lu, M., et al. (2020). "Another tool for the toolbox? I'll take it!": Feasibility and acceptability of mobile recovery outreach teams (MROT) for opioid overdose patients in the emergency room. *Journal of Substance Abuse Treatment, 108*, 95–103.

Waisbord, S. (2001). *Family tree of theories, methodologies and strategies in development communication*. www.comminit.com/?q = global/node/1547

Wallerstein, J. S., & Blakeslee, S. (1990). *Second chances*. Corgi.

Walmart's Opioid Stewardship Initiative. (2018). *Know the facts*. https://corporate.walmart.com/know-the-facts

Ward, J., Hall, W., & Mattick, R. P. (1999). Role of maintenance treatment in opioid dependence. *The Lancet, 353*(9148), 221–226. https://doi.org/10.1016/S0140-6736(98)05356-2

Weick, K. R. (1979). *The social psychology of organizing* (2nd ed.). McGraw-Hill.

Weiser, B., & Thomas, K. (2018, Mar. 16). *5 doctors are charged with taking kickbacks for Fentanyl prescriptions.* The New York Times. https://www.nytimes.com/2018/03/16/nyregion/fentanyl-subsys-drug-kickbacks.html

Wetherell, M., Taylor, S., & Yates, S. J. (Eds.). (2001). *Discourse theory and practice: A reader*. Sage.

White, R. (2016, Sept. 29). *Opioid epidemic's youngest victims are a growing group, new data show*. Center for Health Journalism, University of South Carolina. www.centerforhealthjournalism.org/2016/09/28/opioid-epidemics-youngest-victims-are-growing-group-new-data-show

Wilce, J. M. (2009). Medical discourse. *Annual Review of Anthropology, 38*, 199–215. https://doi.org/10.1146/annurev-anthro-091908-164450

Winter, T., & Schapiro, R. (2019, May 14). *Pennsylvania sues Oxycontin maker Purdue Pharma, says it targeted elderly and vets*. https://www.nbcnews.com/news/us-news/pennsylvania-sues-oxycontin-maker-purdue-pharma-says-it-targeted-elderly-n1005586

Wysowski, D. K., Swann, J., & Vega, A. (2002). Use of isotretinoin (Accutane) in the United States: Rapid increase from 1992 through 2000. *Journal of the American Academy of Dermatology, 46*(4), 505–509. https://doi.org/10.1067/mjd.2002.120529

Yazdy, M. M., Desai, R. J., & Brogly, S. B. (2015). Prescription opioids in pregnancy and birth outcomes: A review of the literature. *Journal of Pediatric Genetics*, *4*(2), 56–70. https://doi.org/10.1055/s-0035-1556740

Yazdy, M. M., Mitchell, A. A., Tinker, S. C., Parker, S. E., & Werler, M. M. (2013). Periconceptional use of opioids and the risk of neural tube defects. *Obstetric and Gynecology*, *122*(4), 838–844. doi:10.1097/AOG.0b013e3182a6643c

Index

About the Author

Rachel Sussman Kaplan, PhD, is an assistant teaching professor of corporate communication at Penn State University Fayette. Her research interests lie at the intersection of health communication, crisis communication, and the marketplace. She has published on the opioid crisis, corporate social responsibility, and Walmart's opioid stewardship initiative. Kaplan is the program coordinator of Corporate Communication and the co-director of the Fayette LaunchBox, a business incubator on campus. She graduated from Duquesne University (PhD), Indiana University of Pennsylvania (MBA), Carlow University (MEd), and the University of Pittsburgh (BA). Kaplan and her husband Richard live with their three wonderful children in Pittsburgh, PA.

www.ingramcontent.com/pod-product-compliance
Ingram Content Group UK Ltd.
Pitfield, Milton Keynes, MK11 3LW, UK
UKHW041839031026
15587UKWH00002B/886

9 781793 640543